Return to Food

Library and Archives Canada Cataloguing in Publication

Strong, Sherry, 1967-, author
    Return to food : the life-changing anti-diet / Sherry Strong.

Issued in print and electronic formats.
ISBN 978-1-77141-060-1 (pbk.).--ISBN 978-1-77141-096-0 (html)

    1. Nutrition. I. Title.

RA784.S89 2014   613.2   C2014-906508-6
                                       C2014-906509-4

RETURN TO FOOD

THE LIFE-CHANGING ANTI-DIET

SHERRY STRONG

Book Cover Design: Marla Thompson
Portrait Photographer: Nino Ellison and Redcity Network
Editing Team: Nina Shoroplova, Steph VanderMeulen, and Susan Kehoe
Typeset: Greg Salisbury

DISCLAIMER: This book has been created to inform individuals with an interest in taking back control of their own health. It is not intended in any way to replace other professional health care or nutritional advice, but to support it. Readers of this publication agree that neither Sherry Strong nor her publisher will be held responsible or liable for damages that may be alleged or resulting, directly, or indirectly, from their use of this publication. All external links are provided as a resource only and are not guaranteed to remain active for any length of time. Neither the publisher nor the author can be held accountable for the information provided by, or actions resulting from accessing these resources. All opinions in this book are those of the author.

disclaimer

this book is based on observing nature & the planet. The Nature Principle is a guiding principle & concept to help people develope a healthy relationship & understanding of .... food

Due to the cheeky nature of the author... pages may contain spelling liberties, controversial thoughts innocent omissions & remarks designed to provoke thought.

*Please read with a generous mind & open heart (not literally an open heart, of course)

dedication

to my parents Jan & Gene who raised me in the culinary equivalent to a gastronomic... black hole *seriously bad food* which provided the perfect environment for rebellion towards nature...

The amazing energy & gifts of the universe for creating this wonderful planet we live in & on.

Thank you Mom & Dad for your amazing love... I am so grateful

TESTIMONIALS

"What I love about this approach is that she has these philosophies, strategies and concepts that just make sense. They help you reframe your thinking in a way that motivates you from the inside. She gives you the tools to tell yourself what to do and in a way that you don't feel like you're missing out."
Theo Fleury, NHL Hockey Legend and Best Selling Author

"It's not an understatement to say that Sherry Strong helped resurrect my life and my health. Her principles within Return To Food illuminate her teachings, which should be required reading for anyone interested in lifelong health, energy, and normalizing body weight. This is not a diet; it's reclaiming your natural right to eat the way you were designed to eat."
Jon Benson, CEO, Sellerator.com, Creator of The Video Sales Letter

"Sherry Strong is more than her impressive list of achievements in the nutrition world that include sitting as Victorian Chair of Nutrition Australia and sought after lecturer at IHN, one of our most prestigious nutrition schools in the country. She is, as her title so eloquently describes, "a food philosopher" who cares deeply about her students. This book is a goldmine resource for anyone who wants to cut out the crap and get healthy once and for all."
Sheleana Breakell & Caleb Jennings, Co-Founders, YoungandRaw.com

"(Sherry) has really made it so understandable, how being simple and eating food that is good for you is actually returning to nature, and we love that philosophy – it is our philosophy!"
Mariel Hemingway & Bobby Williams, Authors of Running With Nature

"Sherry gets that I have an extremely active and busy life that doesn't fit into a cookie cutter quick fix prescriptive approach. She tailors her work to suit my life. Her concepts and philosophies make complex and conflicting information make sense so I can apply her practical wisdom into my way of doing life."
W. Brett Wilson, Entrepreneur, Philanthropist & 3-Season Panelist on CBC's Dragons' Den

"Sherry's knowledge on the subject of health is extensive...(her) passion is abundant and it's a pleasure to work with her. Best decision I have EVER made...eternally grateful."
Debra Ross, CEO, Gamma Tech

"Sherry is one of the world's most lucid experts in the area of food and nutrition."
Taren Hocking, Champion Events

"The nutritional guidance I have received from Sherry has enabled me, at the age of 50, to operate at a peak I couldn't have even imagined in my 20s. Best of all I enjoy how I source, store, prepare, share and ingest beautiful, natural foods. Her holistic approach to wellness works for me on so many levels."
Jan Saunders, Elite Athlete & Endurance Event Competitor

Acknowledgements

This book has been an evolutionary project, twenty-plus years in the making. I knew I didn't want to do a cookbook, but that there was a book in me. After ten years of talking and planning, and more talking and writing, friends politely stopped asking where the book was. Thank you to all of you who gave me that grace. The book has been supported by too many people to mention here, many of whom may not know they were integral to my process, and more who I'm sure have helped in ways that have just not come to me right now.

My dearest friend Helen inspired me when I hand wrote and illustrated her life story in a beautiful green clothbound book for her fortieth birthday. Helen showed it to her husband, David, an amazing, prolific author, who suggested to her that it would be a great format for my philosophies. This started my love of illustrating the things I'm passionate about. I showed the first illustrations to Tim Smith of Books for Cooks in Melbourne, who suggested I accompany the illustrations with more "gravitas," the definition of which I had to go home and look up. Thus began the creation and research of a great deal of supporting information that was compiled over almost eight years.

Thank you to Julie Salisbury, my publisher (and her wonderful team), who allowed me to keep the copyright to my philosophies and illustrations with the Influence business model. To Steph, for your incredible passionate commitment to editing the book so more people would be able to devour it. To Olga, for finding Steph and providing insight into my need to refine the book, as well as for our fabulous friendship.

For the hundreds of friends on Facebook who provided feedback for covers and illustrations over the years. For all the clients who've provided testimonials and allowed me to use their story to help others: Marie, Jordan, Theo, Debra, Tim, and Brett. Thank you to the students who've supported my work and allowed me to do what I love.

To Callie, who provided me with a soulmate love that only a mother could experience. I miss you, my dear sweet soul, and am grateful for all those mornings you sat on my lap as the sweetest loving muse anyone could ask for, my angel baby girl. To Billy, for your grumpy love button meows, lap cuddles, and staying with me after Callie passed.

Thank you to my parents for love and support that exceeds what a child has any right to expect, not to mention a belief in me that exceeded how I could see myself. Thank you for never letting me forget it. DJ, my love and soulmate. You are supportive beyond words I have the capacity to express. Your belief in me and this work never fails to amaze me. I am so very grateful to share this journey with you. Thank you, my love.

To the Universe and the network of awesome that connects us all. I am in awe and humbled by how you work. Thank you for showing me that if I can believe in my dreams and take a step each day to follow them, amazing things happen, beautiful things show up.

Lastly, to everyone who picks up this book and reads it, and tells a friend and shares the philosophies or a recipe over dinner. Thank you for being part of a revolution that has the power to change your life and save our beautiful planet.

Bless you all.
With love,
Sherry

Contents

Foreword

When Bobby and I first met Sherry, we connected over her illustrations, which captured and showed us she really got the philosophies we live by.

Through subsequent visits and sharing meals in each other's homes in California and Melbourne, Australia, we saw that we also share a world view, a way of being that is not about dieting or depriving yourself of food but simply eating real food as close to nature as you can possibly get.

We have become a society that eats to fill up, to satisfy cravings that have nothing to do with nourishment. Food is often mistaken for a way to achieve love, comfort, and understanding. We eat out of boredom, fear, complacency, and apathy or out of a lack of feeling what we feel in our bodies. Food has become a way to anesthetize and cover our hurts.

For years, my partner Bobby William's parents said that how he ate (which was pure and simple; raw, sprouted, and live food) was alternative, and that he wasn't living in reality. Only recently, when they got turned onto eating simple food themselves, did they say, "Oh, I get it … now that I feel so much better, I see that we thought you were alternative when in fact it is everyone else who eats alternatively. You eat real food, the way nature intended us to eat." In their retired years, they are discovering the beauty of their food, and their good health and happiness are the result.

It is my passion, as well as Bobby's and Sherry's, to reveal the power of nature, in all its simplicity and purity, in food. It is not about a new diet: it is about balance and finding a way to eat that speaks to your personal body and spirit. It is about making loving choices that are kind, simple, and right for you.

I personally have been a follower of every diet. I have been vegan (fourteen years), vegetarian, and macrobiotic. I ate fruit for a year along with a lot of Espresso. I was a raw vegan as well (very gassy year!), and now, finally, I have come to eating just clean, simple, real food. I eat animal protein only when it is not abused. I also eat organic and biodynamic fruits and vegetables whenever possible.

My choices are influenced by my love of the power of food. It has the ability to lift me up into a state of pure delight or sink me into sadness. I suffered depression years ago and came to the realization that food is like a drug, and the simpler and cleaner I ate, the simpler, cleaner mind and happier thoughts I had. I can prevent mood swings, depression, and terror with what I ingest. I spent a great deal of my life trying to survive it, and part of my survival was eating obsessively. The outcome of extreme dieting or overindulgence in toxic food made me a fearful girl and woman. That is no longer a part of my life. In fact, now food is part of my connection to self, nature, and God.

As Sherry will tell you, eating is a celebration of the senses. It is a ritual that makes us LIVE on a deep level. Food can be our medicine; it can be our joy and our healing, and every bit of it can be a spiritual experience. We are here to experience the joy of food. We honour food by growing it ourselves if possible, by picking it, choosing it, preparing it with gentle hands, and being aware of the consciousness that food holds.

When I had my daughters I became aware that what I ingested was profoundly important to the development of my babies. It was amazing to think that when I nursed them, I was giving them food that I created myself. I knew that if I ate the purest food, that nourishment would help them develop into healthy strong and happy people.

Real food is not a science project; it is a product of nature's expression of love. It is an expression of beauty, energy, and growth in combination with the rest of nature, the sun, water, and air. It is the outcome of nature's power to provide for all creatures great and small.

Bobby and I live by the philosophies Sherry shares in Return to Food. They really are grounded in nature, and now in our fifties we feel more alive and vibrant than ever.

We hope you enjoy Return to Food and dip into the philosophies and recipes with the same soulful intention with which Sherry has created them. They are not only delicious, but they truly have the power to change your life.

Mariel Hemingway

Mariel is not only an Oscar-nominated actress but the author of several books on food, nutrition, and holistic living. *Running with Nature* was cowritten with her partner in love and life, Bobby Williams, who is also an actor, stuntman, and nutritionist.

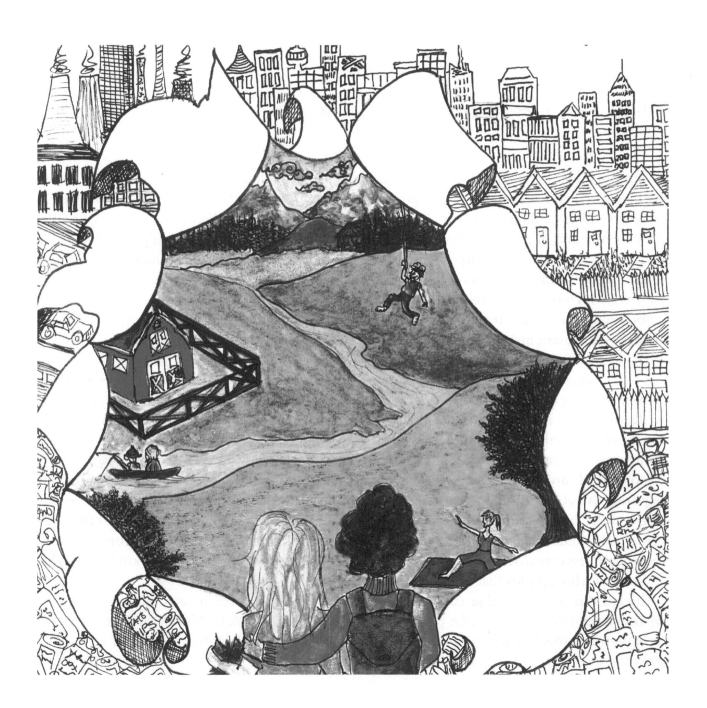

INTRODUCTION

Why Going Back Is the Way Forward

This is not a diet book. The intention of this book is to debunk the myth that you need to diet to get healthy. Therefore, you won't find prescriptive measures, formulas, or strategies to lose weight or reverse disease, though many of my clients have become fit and disease-free by adopting the philosophies and principles I offer here to help you develop a healthy relationship with food, your body, and the planet. These philosophies are designed to help you understand how you are meant to eat—not according to my way of eating, but by listening, observing, and respecting the messages your body is constantly conveying to you.

Food is so much more than fuel for the body and pleasure for the palate. Labelling it exclusively as such is a reductionist model that has a world swaying from indulgence to denial. We've lost the amazing, beautiful experience that eating and nurturing our entire being can be. Food can nourish the body, please the palate, enrich the soul, create connection, and satisfy hunger, among other things. Ignoring even one of these aspects limits the awareness and depth of our experience. When we learn how to nurture our amazing body with mental, emotional, spiritual, and physical food worthy of our souls, real change occurs. Finding meaningful connection in how we feed our being always seems to carry over into a more meaningful, vibrant, loving life.

Most people are surprised to learn they are not eating real food. Determining what real food is requires navigation, intuition, holistic vision, and sometimes patience. But I've seen miracles occur simply with the act of returning to eating real food. Weight loss is minor compared to the body being truly nourished, sometimes for the first time in their life. I've seen healing go on not just in the body to reverse disease symptoms, but also in the heart, in simply choosing kinder thoughts and more loving options that nourish the body inside out.

Though this is not a cookie-cutter, one-size-fits-all approach, there are commonalties between what does and does not work for people. The first part of this book is about what is not working, an experiment that has gone wrong. The latter part of the book is about how we can turn it around, one meal at a time.

There is no one way for all to return to food. This is your own unique journey of well-being and finding what you need and want, and what works best for you with regard to the philosophies in this book.

Return to Food is about a return to loving our body and our planet without judgment and with an open heart and mind. I urge you to consume these words in a gentle, mindful way, to digest every bite of the information, knowledge, and wisdom with a spoonful of love, so you get this approach intellectually as well as take it into your heart.

This book urges you not to wait for scientific proof of the damaging effects of processed foods. There are plenty already, and so many of them contradict each other. There is no need to depend on them. Trust me on this. If you are ready to listen to your body—the amazing, intuitive creature it is—you will instinctively understand how you should eat. I will show you how this works.

And the result? As I said: diet no longer needed. You are free to be yourself.

The Diet Mentality

For years I tried many different diets, only to end up worse off than I was before I started. After disturbingly gaining eight sizes, I came to the conclusion that others have also discovered: dieting does not work. The diet mentality has reduced our relationship with food to being about weight loss, which goes against the natural purpose of physical nourishment. Our relationship with food is not meant to be about restriction, obsession, weighing ourselves and our food, and focusing on what we cannot have. This pattern of behaviour and thought is greatly responsible for the widespread dysfunction in our relationship with food, our bodies, and the planet, and we need to turn it around quickly for our health care system, our environment, and our own quality of life.

The prescriptive approach to food, often contradictory and constantly changing, has led to an epidemic of confusion about what to eat. In addition, it's become increasingly difficult to navigate the overwhelming world of processed, chemically laden food. Transitioning to a real food diet can take years to figure out on your own. The purpose of this book is to get you there faster, using the framework and details I use to help clients through lifestyle makeovers.

I want you to develop a healthy, stress-free, and joy-filled relationship with food, your body, and the planet. It is my hope you will share this with your circle of influence, as a leader, coach, or advocate.

When I poll audiences in corporate presentations, I ask, "Who experiences nutritional confusion, when one day you hear a certain food is the healthiest thing you can eat and another day you hear that it is dangerous and to be avoided?" Usually, about 40 percent of the people raise their hands. But when I poll recent nutrition graduates with the same question, about 90 percent raise their hands. Greater knowledge does not always lead to clarity.

Today, we are drowning in a deluge of nutritional information, created by a plague of convincing nutrition gurus who are convinced they have found the way for you. The problem is, their beliefs are often at odds. How can you possibly know what is right and, in particular, right for you? With *Return to Food*, I hope to help clarify this for you.

In Chapter One, I share some of my personal journey through dieting, weight gain, depression, my tumultuous relationship with food, and my eventual understanding of true health. I also talk about the prevalent misconceptions about weight loss and healthy eating, and outline my answer to the epidemics of obesity and disease—my Return to Food approach.

The philosophies and concepts shared in Chapters Two, Three, and Four are designed to cut through the nutritional confusion and offer you clarity about how it is *you* are designed to be eating, so you are never at the mercy of nutritional marketing and media manipulation.

Knowledge is good, but in order to make long-term sustainable changes, we require wisdom to reach a new level of awareness. We need to look at ourselves in a holistic sense—that is, we are mental, emotional, spiritual, and physical beings—and apply that belief to the way we take care of ourselves.

Chapter Five discusses a tool I've intuitively used for years but only recently put into practice as a process. It is one of the key aspects of the anti-diet mentality and why the subtitle of this book—"The Life-Changing Anti-Diet"— is most relevant. When you focus on nourishing all four quadrants of your being—the physical, emotional, spiritual, and mental—the food side of things will begin to take care of itself, making dieting obsolete.

In Chapter Six, I talk about a universal recipe for healing that works for all humans once they start listening to their body and determining what they need. In Chapter Seven, I go beyond food to self-love and self-care. This is absolutely essential, the most important nutrient, to the *Return to Food* approach. I ask you to consider how significant love is in relation to our nourishment and healing, and give you tips for how to be kind to and nurture yourself and others through connection, food, and holistic well-being.

In Chapter Eight, I bring together all the previous philosophies and concepts to help you create your own Life Kitchen, full of the tools and ingredients needed to set you on the holistic path and return you to eating real food.

Although this is not a diet book, the next section contains recipes for you to try so you can sample what real food is and have ideas for moving forward on your own. These recipes use only natural and beneficial foods. They've been tested for nutritional value, taste, and ease. Enjoy!

Over the past fourteen years, I've noticed a common path for those on their journey to health. As a result, in the Epilogue I show you the Holistic Hero's Journey. With this, you can decide where you are on the path, where you've been, and how to get to a place of true peace around food and eating.

Return to Food is about how to nourish yourself in a way that is joyful, sustainable, and lasting. It goes beyond the physical aspects of ourselves and shows you how to avoid toxicity and move beyond basic nutrition to "HyperNourishing" yourself (explained in Chapter Five), in nonfood ways that compel you to make better choices naturally. It reveals what is happening to our food and how we can return to eating real food, the kind that sustains, protects, and energizes us while creating a stronger planet in the process.

To succeed at *Return to Food*, you have to be able to distinguish between what is real food and what is not, get access to and find real food, and learn how to prepare and eat what once was normal. This is now tricky, but I want to make the process of returning to food as simple as possible for you. I'm not suggesting it is the easiest path—our desire for ease, thinking it will make us happy, is part of the reason we have such a messed-up food system. "Ease" is relative, and the effort you invest up front, I assure you, will pay dividends in better health, happiness, energy levels, mental acuity, and mood balance. I will show you how.

This book does not have to be read in a specific order, though for it to make sense as a process, I do recommend it. However, if you like, you can skip ahead to the Universal Recipe for Healing, in Chapter 6, or to the recipes that follow Chapter Eight, if you're eager to give them a try. Whichever way you decide to read Return to Food, may it guide you to holistic well-being and happiness.

Chapter One

The Cost of Fast and Easy

An All-Too-Common Story—With an Uncommon Twist

I wasn't always strong by name or nature. I was born a sickly, sensitive baby. I never suckled my mother's milk, because she was convinced by doctors and nurses that baby formula was better. Fed this formula—made of what I now call "the Lethal Recipe," that is, refined sugars, refined oils, refined salts, refined grains, and refined chemicals including MSG, a known neurotoxin—I became the perfect candidate for addiction to processed food and, as a result, for illnesses, obesity, and disease. For much of my infancy, I was sick and malnourished.

Like millions of others, perhaps even you, I grew up a fan of what looked, smelled, and tasted like food but in fact was not. As a child, I used to collect pop bottles to get change to feed my sugar addiction. I'd buy Double Bubble gum and Mojos for a few cents, and steal Tang, the tart and sweet juice powder, from the cupboard to blissfully eat in hiding. I loved cooking anything with sugar in it and always wanted to bake. My Easy Bake Oven was the greatest gift ever.

At that time, of course I made no connection between my eating and the terrible effects of the withdrawal; I didn't know I was already an addict.

During my childhood, most of the food we ate was highly processed and came out of packets and boxes. The vegetables (with the rare exception of those from gardens we raided or were allowed to take from) were from a supermarket, conventionally farmed, and cooked to their death. Even worse were tinned vegetables that were dead to start with and boiled long just in case they had not been preserved correctly.

Much of the food in my childhood felt deeply unsatisfying. For my hyperstimulated, chemically addicted palate and body, whole foods were boring. Super-flavoured foods were the only ones that seemed to register interest, with very few exceptions. I remember my grandmother taking me to my great-grandmother's home for lunch. She had made a soup, something like beef barley, and I could see the bones in it, which disturbed me. I hesitated to try it. After much convincing, I reluctantly took a mouthful. My eyes widened; this was a culinary awakening for me. I'd never tasted soup like this before. It was delicious and real. Campbell and Heinz had never made anything like it. I remember the room erupted with laughter when I asked for another bowl.

Nevertheless, processed foods remained the staples of my diet. My teen years were riddled with depression, hypoglycemia, terribly painful menses, sinus infections, a dreadful body image, and migraine headaches, much of which I did not grow out of until I weaned myself off of food that wasn't serving me.

In the late 1980s, I moved to Australia from Canada, met a man in Melbourne, married, and became a chef. It was as if I'd been given a professional excuse to overeat and stuff down my feelings. Now in my twenties, my food addiction had increased to the point where I was obese, struggling to fit into pants eight sizes larger than I presently wear. I used food to avoid feeling uncomfortable and to celebrate anything that felt good, hoping the feeling would last longer. Of course, it didn't. The food hangovers were so bad that the only thing I could do to feel better was eat, and you can bet it wasn't broccoli I was looking for, unless it was covered in copious amounts of cheese sauce.

Being a career chef in a commercial kitchen didn't appeal to me, so instead I founded a cooking school called The Foodlovers Workshop. Ironically, I ran Low-Fat Classes at a time when I was drastically overweight. I always wondered if students thought I ate any of my low-fat dishes or if they thought I ate all of them.

The classes were popular, because I never used low-fat, fake-fat anything. They came to the attention of dietitian Theo O'Conner, who introduced me to Dr. Rick Kausman, author of *If Not Dieting, Then What?* (2005). Rick turned my attention to Nutrition Australia, an organization that educates the public on matters of nutritional well-being. After a year on the committee, I was appointed Chair for Nutrition Australia for the State of Victoria. This was an eye-opening time for me, as I discovered the degree to which food politics operates in the nutrition world and how it impacts what we eat and what we believe is healthy for us.

I decided to study nutrition at Deakin University, which opened my eyes even more to the influence of the food industry on the curricula of schools and the biases that are developed by students who don't question their own indoctrination. At the time, the system seemed to be preparing an army of people trained and credentialed to espouse the goodness of a conventional food system funded by the food industry.

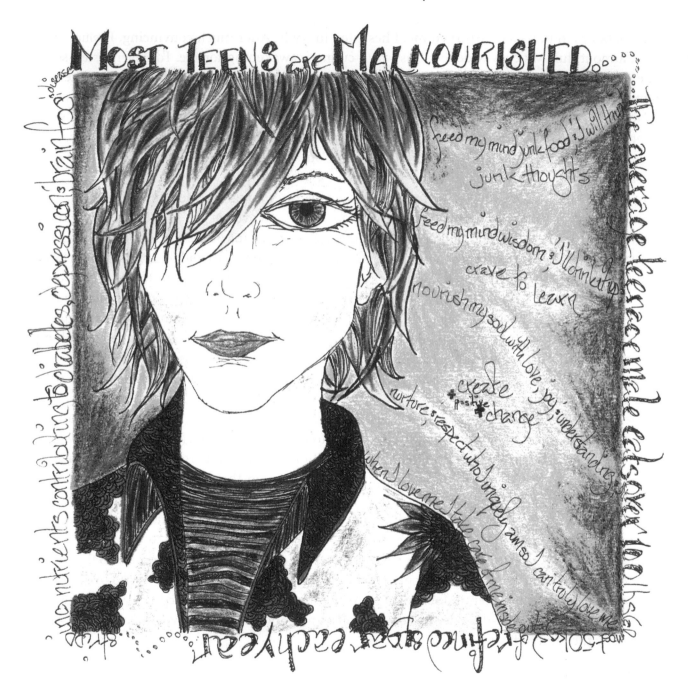

MOST TEENS are MALNOURISHED...

feed my mind junk food & I will think junk thoughts

feed my mind wisdom & I'll think up crave to learn

nourish my soul with love, joy, understanding

create positive change

nurture & respect who I am so I can truly love me

when I love me I take care of me inside & out

The average teenage male eats over 100 lbs of...

...of sugar each year!

...no nutrients contributing to diabetes, depression & brain fog

Millions of people are needlessly sick, tired, and dying because of our miseducation. And I was one of them. In 1996, I was twice my present size. I was angry at life, taking it out on my husband and colleagues. Headaches, migraines, back pain, depression, nausea, heartburn, regular bouts of colds and flu, asthma, and acne were just some of my ailments the drugs in my medicine cabinet treated.

I remember one morning vividly, when I awoke with a massive hangover (despite not having consumed alcohol). Although I'd slept eight hours, I felt as though thirty more would not have been enough. I didn't want to hit the snooze button—I wanted to blast my alarm clock into smithereens with a sledgehammer. I rolled over in bed and watched my stomach follow and roll onto the bed like a sack filled with jelly. I sat up in bed feeling miserable, sad, and incredibly frustrated, trapped in a body of my own doing, wondering, "How have I managed to do this? How bad is it going to get before I do something?" Stepping into the shower that morning, avoiding the mirrors, I grabbed the handfuls of flesh and cried out in frustration as the warm water beat down on my face, carrying my tears away down the drain.

I got dressed in the size 14 pants that were too tight. I'd been too proud to buy the size 16 pair I'd tried on earlier that week. I could not face that humiliation; for me, owning them meant I was comfortable with that size, and I was not.

That day I reached the threshold. Enough was enough. I would figure this out. I would unlock the key of why I—a chef, nutritionist, and student of nutrition for half my life at that point—was eating all this food I knew was making me fat and creating ailments that demanded I fill my medicine cabinet with treatments that did nothing to address their cause.

The truth is I was your average overweight neighbour, colleague, sister, daughter, wife, and woman wanting a better life in a better body, and wanting it so badly—so desperately—that I was willing to do anything to lose that weight, except change what I was eating and move my butt off the couch. I wanted a quick fix, a pill, a potion, some magic trick that would have the weight fall off overnight, and I set out to find it.

Of course, I never did find a quick fix that was legit. I found lots of things that were marketed well, concepts of weight loss gurus that, if I could follow their unnatural restrictive plans, promised I would lose the weight. I tried everything out there, and when I'd exhausted that, I came up with my own ideas and experiments, which in the end always failed. Sometimes, I lost weight, but I looked older and more stressed and felt flat and tired all the time. Ultimately, the weight piled back on.

I spent thousands of dollars to discover that nothing worked. It was only when I finally tried the thing I feared most that things started to turn around. And when I saw the success that came from that, I began to explore the next logical and sometimes counterintuitive move, based on what I had seen work in other people and other cultures.

After a long struggle and a new approach to health, things are different now. Today, I get out of bed with energy, motivation, and mental clarity. I don't visit drug stores or chemists anymore; I can't even remember the last time I needed a prescription from a doctor.

I finally got to this stage without dieting or drugs. Through trial and error, I discovered that the best agent for healing the body is the body. When you give the body what it needs to heal itself, it does so remarkably well. And what we need most does not come from a packet, a bottle, or an injection, but directly from the earth and the sun. I also learned that we are far more than simply physical beings bound by what we feed on and how we move; how we think and feel also affects our wellness.

Now I live a life that years ago I could not have imagined. I travel the world giving talks about the philosophies behind *Return to Food*. I am a consultant to professional athletes, celebrities, and CEOs. I've worked with youth at risk through foundations started by Jamie Oliver and the Australian football legend, Jim Stynes. I teach future educators how to instruct at the Institute of Holistic Nutrition in Vancouver, British Columbia, and at my own Return to Food Academy.

After twenty-one years, I've come to see how emotional wellness impacts what and how we eat and how we think and feel. I've also seen this pattern in many clients. This experience may be resonating with you right now as well. If so, you are not alone. I wrote this book for you.

Why Diets Don't Work

Anger, shame, and judgment aren't likely to make anyone feel bad enough to feel good about doing better.

In general, diets often fail for several reasons: they don't teach people how to live according to natural instinct and intuition; they rely too much on willpower; they sell a solution that is difficult to apply to our daily lives; they indulge their followers by allowing them to eat as much junk as they want so long as they count calories; they don't address the mental and emotional factors that drive us to eat what we eat.

Typically, diets teach you how to measure food, count calories, or assign points to the food you eat. They condition you to measure success based on numbers, not on how well you are nourished, how you feel, how much energy you have, or any true measure of health. Scales do not measure how big or healthy your heart is or the goodness in your heart. They can't show what a giving, caring, loving, and intelligent person you are, or measure your wisdom, your worth, or your contribution to the planet.

Diets have it all figured out for you. They simply tell you what to do. In other words, they give you a fish rather than have you pay attention to your intelligence, intuition, and instinct so you can catch that fish yourself. Diets disregard the great wisdom of nature and what it provides and has provided for millennia to keep us healthy and fit.

When I first started telling clients what they should and shouldn't eat, their success was limited. I was frustrated and confused; after all, it made so much sense. But when I started to work more intuitively with people, getting them to listen to and trust their own bodies, they progressed significantly. When I started to use the philosophical approach, they understood the relationship to food on a deeper level and learned for themselves what it was they were meant to be eating, how much, and when. Next, I realized that doing the inner work was key to lasting wellness, weight loss, and disease-symptom reversal.

> *"You cannot solve a problem from the same consciousness that created it.*
> *You must learn to see the world anew."*
> **Albert Einstein**

Over a period of ten years, I developed methods to help people work on their "MindSet" and "HeartSet," vital pieces to the puzzle of why we eat the way we do. Unless a person has the MindSet and HeartSet pieces in place, they will eventually return to old patterns of behaviour, eating the types and amounts of food that got them sick, fat, and tired to begin with.

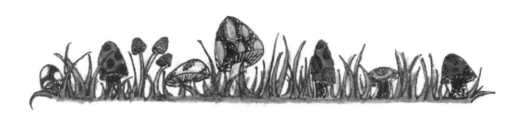

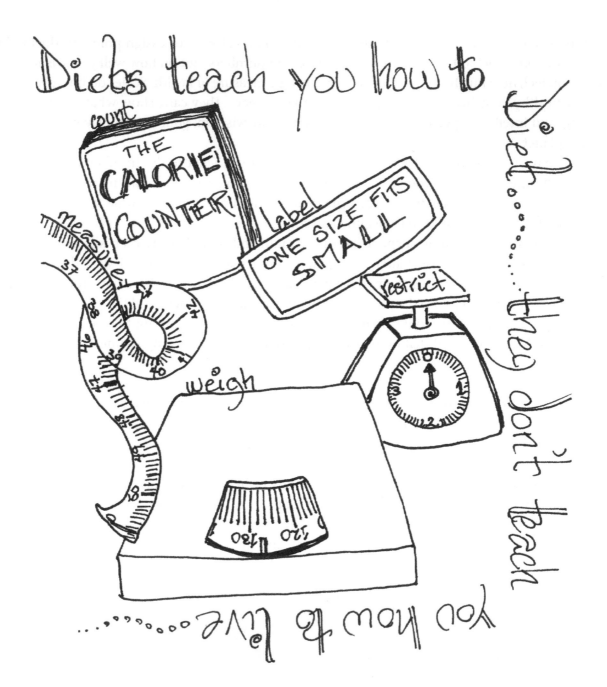

Diets teach you how to

count

THE
CALORIE
COUNTER!

measure

37

38

39

40

label

ONE SIZE FITS
SMALL

restrict

weigh

Diet.........they don't teach

you how to live.........

Aided by my discoveries and fuelled by personal success, I began to work more closely with clients, getting into their kitchens, shopping for them, creating what I call a "Life Kitchen," combined with all the modalities detailed in this book. Eventually, my approach drew the attention of former NHL star Theo Fleury, who for years had been plagued with pain that doctors could not relieve. After following my program, Theo lost forty pounds and reversed his symptoms of Crohn's disease. I was also privileged to work with W. Brett Wilson, a panelist on CBC's Dragons' Den, who applied my anti-diet approach, learned to develop a healthier relationship with food, and brought his whole family into my kitchen for classes. Socialite CEO Debra Ross—a beautiful bachelorette with an empty fridge and gut issues to go with it—experienced her own health transformation after following my program. Andrew, another CEO, came to me with newly diagnosed diabetes and a diet from his doctor that was designed to keep him on insulin. After only one week of working with me, all his diabetic symptoms disappeared.

Many more clients have experienced seemingly miraculous transformations, as long as they've stuck with the food, and even without access to the resources and influence of the people above. Well-being has little to do with resources. When you find the *why* of your lifestyle, the way forward will present itself.

If we just went back to the way we ate 100 years ago, we'd halve lifestyle diseases in a year; progress can absolutely be obtained without technological advances. The thought that technology with regard to our food system has contributed significantly to modern day lifestyle diseases is counter intuitive in a world brainwashed to believe technology is the answer to everything that ails us. Though rarely a sexy or lucrative solution, sometimes the answer is going back.

THE BIGGEST EATING DISORDER

In 2009, after finding out what I do for a living, the man sitting next to me on a plane asked what I thought of *The Biggest Loser* television show. I went on a bit of a rant, starting with, "You mean the Biggest Eating Disorder?" I went on to explain how the show was creating an unhealthy, fat-phobic culture, and how the practice of "game-ifying" eating was detrimental to our well-being, and perpetuated exactly the opposite of what the show claimed to promote.

At that point, I looked up and, mortified, saw he was wearing a *Biggest Loser* baseball cap. Turns out he was one of the casting directors. But he acknowledged a few points I'd made and said I wasn't the first to express them.

Eating is nowadays portrayed as a punishment one moment, a treat another. It's shown as binging. It involves pitting people against each other, comparing, manipulating, tempting, and bribing. Quick weight loss at any cost and means, overtraining with heavy weights, seclusion from reality, enormous external pressure for validation and reward—all of these perpetuate the same unhealthy mentality that creates disordered eating. The truth is that what works does not make for sensational television and lucrative advertising. The solution does not lie in contests or deprivation, but in something much deeper and grounded.

Even the strictest health advocates can have eating issues if they make their choices out of fear and loathing instead of love. If they are primarily motivated by fear of disease or getting fat, rather than by moving toward well-being, there will be imbalance. They will not be healthy or vibrant.

Return to Food Revolution of Love and Evolution

*A weight loss is not always a health gain. You can be just as unhealthy in a thin
body as in an overweight body.*

People are often surprised to find out that in my work as a nutritionist I see many clients who are not overweight, but still suffer from diabetes, cancer, heart disease, and other lifestyle illnesses. The irony of their situation is that they are in some cases at a higher risk for disease even though they are slim. Let me explain.

*Don't judge a book by its cover; disordered eating comes in bodies of all shapes
and sizes.*

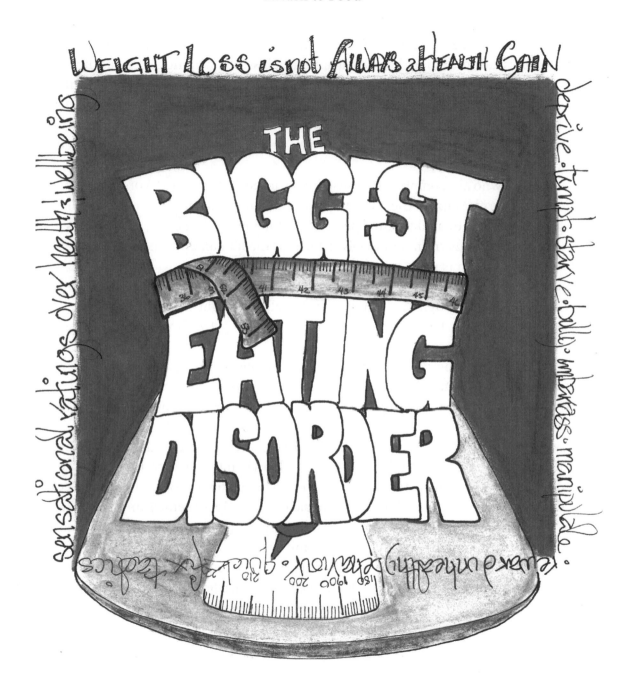

The body creates fat cells to store excess energy, but fat has all kinds of protective functions, like guarding nerve tissue, insulating the body against heat loss, and helping to regulate hormonal functions. The body will also create fat cells to store excess toxins to keep them away from vital organs. If you are working strategically to keep your fat levels below what is necessary for good health, while eating a low-calorie diet of nutrient-deficient, chemically laden products (which includes many weight-loss products and supplements), your vital organs are at risk of being affected by excess toxins via your blood.

I've seen people who are completely, unsustainably unhealthy go to extraordinary lengths to lose weight and keep fat off. Many of them have been featured in magazines and in the media for getting their weight or fat down to an unnatural percentile, oblivious to the cost to their bodies. Eating real food—that is, whole foods from nature—is critical for the human body, no matter what size or the amount of fat. Being thin is not a cure for disease.

I've lost weight both through clean eating and pure caloric restriction, where I got down to a weight that sent terror through me. I felt like I was walking a tightwire, because I knew I could not sustain that way of eating. It was too restrictive and it didn't gel with what or how I really felt like eating.

When I lost weight eating whole foods, my body radiated and was firm, but when I simply restricted calories and continued to eat processed food, my body was thinner, but my complexion was drawn and my skin did not bounce back firmly when pressed even lightly. I looked older and I was still not healthy.

My first encounter with clean eating came not long after leaving high school, when I read a book called *Fit for Life* (1985), by Harvey and Marilyn Diamond, which first educated me about processed food. I tried to follow its guidance, but on a student budget of ten dollars a week for food, the two-dollar-a-piece avocados that were a staple of the recipes seemed impossible to fund. The actual diet was so far from my processed diet that even though it made sense and resonated on a certain level, it was too much for me to aspire to and sustain. I knew that for something to work for me, it couldn't be a diet, because everything within me hates restriction.

I didn't know it then, but in hindsight the whole process needed to be more organic (not just the food), and that became the approach that I grew into. I had made eating about being thin, but it was so much more than that, as we will explore in this book.

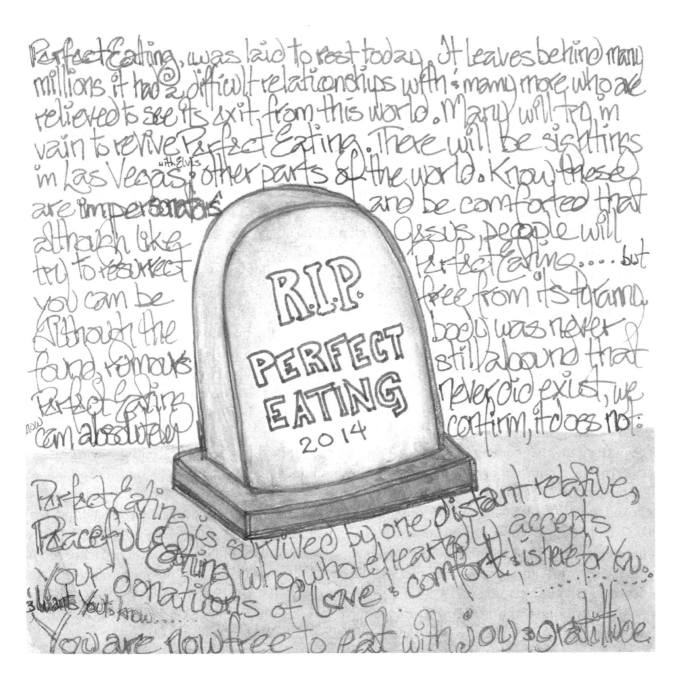

Perfect Eating, was laid to rest today. It leaves behind many millions it had a difficult relationships with, many more who are relieved to see its exit from this world. Many will try, in vain to revive Perfect Eating. There will be sightings in Las Vegas & other parts of the world. Know these are impersonators, although like with Elvis try to resurrect you can be without the found, famous Perfect Eating now can absolutely

and be comforted that Jesus people will Perfect Eating.... but free from its tyranny. body was never still abound that never did exist, we confirm, it does not.

Perfect Eating is survived by one distant relative, Peaceful Eating who wholeheartedly accepts your donations of love & comfort is there for you. & wants you to know...... You are now free to eat with joy & gratitude.

R.I.P.
PERFECT EATING
2014

RIP Perfect Eating

Before we go any further, I want to get one thing straight: I'm a nutritionist, not the Gandhi, Mother Teresa, Dalai Lama, or Jesus of food. I eat to make myself feel good (in a healthy way)—while I'm eating, after I've eaten, and the next day. But I'm also human: I can eat for pure momentary pleasure, too, even when I know I'm not going to feel so good after or the next morning. Being a nutritionist does not make me immune to food temptation any more than becoming a priest provides immunity against sexual temptation.

Sometimes, I eat chocolate at breakfast time, admittedly only a square or two, not a whole bar. The quality is exceptional. This is a far cry from the days when I'd down half a litre of Sara Lee Ultra Chocolate Ice Cream at breakfast and didn't stop eating all day. For the first thirty-five years of my life, I used food as a way to feel good when inside I felt like screaming, or I was sad, frustrated, and unable to speak my truth. I ate when I was unable to create thoughts that led to better feelings.

But I've come a long way since then. Now, the call for balance comes in the messages my body lovingly screams at me to remind me to return to eating food that benefits me. Now, my choices are healthier, the portions are smaller, and I am more readily bringing myself into consciousness while doing it. My self-talk is much kinder and forgiving, too, these days. Peace comes from an acceptance of where I am, a surrender to what feels like my God-given passion for food, acceptance of the fact that I thoroughly enjoy eating, and I deeply enjoy food in many forms. The last was once testified to by the fact that a guy broke up with me based on how much joy I experienced eating good pizza.

Contrary to what some may think, eating just raw foods is not the only healthy way to eat. It's true that the simple act of cooking food diminishes nutrients and makes the food more addictive. People tend to eat more cooked food than raw. Sound way off base? Pretty hard to swallow that cooked food is "addictive"? Then try giving it up for a year—highly processed and cooked food, that is. To be honest, if someone had suggested the same to me fifteen years ago, I would have laughed them off as a quack. Going without cooking your food (as raw foodists advocate) is tricky. So I'm not saying don't cook any of your food. However, the less you cook and the more raw food you incorporate, the better you will feel.

As a nutritionist, the pressure to eat perfectly can be suffocating. That pressure comes from self-expectations, students, family, clients, and fellow colleagues. I've met people who have pretty close to perfect eating habits and often they feel just as conflicted, which is why the "*Return to Food movement*" is about peace and love generated from within first. I've met angry vegans who've tried to intimidate, bully, and shame people into eating according to their ethics, which frankly I totally respect (the ethics, not the tactics). Often people who've eaten meat for decades become vegan and then condemn others who are simply doing what they did for most of their lives; they expect everyone to "see the light" it took them decades to see. But you cannot shame or bully someone into a more enlightened way of being. As I said before, eating well has to come from a place of love, not fear or stress.

The key to balance is to pick your poisons. You can read more about this in Chapter Four, where I talk about the Consumption Concept.

Nature's Principle

Return to Food has always been based on nature, connecting to nature, and intuitive thinking. It is about being connected to the elements and forces that nourish and energize us as well as protect us from disease.

When I first began to explore the concepts of my anti-diet approach, I put all the pieces of the puzzle together in a way that helped others make sense out of the extreme confusion that exists about what to eat, how to eat, how much to eat, and what is truly good for us.

I was out walking in nature one day when an idea hit me. It was autumn and the leaves were changing but still abundant on the trees. A cool breeze made me pick up my pace a bit. I remember looking up at the trees and a few clouds and asking myself, "How can I teach this and make sense of it all? How and what are we meant to eat?" Then I had an aha moment that was like an intellectual lottery win. It was a concept I've had the privilege to share in numerous countries with people whose lives have been transformed by the sense it makes.

This idea, what I call "Nature's Principle," is based on observing how we interact with our natural environment. I share Nature's Principle with you in detail in Chapter Three, but here I introduce it to you as the foundation of my Return to Food philosophies.

From what I've observed, I've come to believe that nature is far more intelligent and wise than man, and that all we need to solve the problems we've created environmentally are contained within nature. The key lies in the human species working with nature, not fighting it or being at war with our planet.

We don't need to know how nature works in order to know that nature works, just as we don't need to know how to breathe in order to breathe, or how our thought processes work in order to think. The wise way of the future is just to work within the boundaries of nature, mindful that we don't know the long-term ramifications of some things. Poisoning insects that impact the plants we eat and the soil meant to grow future food, and leaching chemicals and contaminants into our waterways, are short-sighted measures. The wisdom of traditional cultures cautions us to tread as lightly as we possibly can.

Consider the wisdom of traditional cultures (which we've also called primitive), like that of the Australian Aboriginals, who lived completely in harmony with nature with little to no impact on their environment. Success in the Australian Aboriginal culture was to maintain an invisible ecological footprint.

It was only after a forceful colonization and reservation system imposed "progressive thinking" on them that they, for the first time in tens of thousands of years, began to have a negative impact on their environment. They adopted the "Lethal Recipe." This was immediately evident as an epidemic increase in lifestyle diseases. When I spoke to a dentist in the northern regions of Australia while I was conducting research, he told me he had over three hundred patients under the age of six in a small Queensland community who required all of their teeth to be pulled; most of the children were of indigenous origins clearly not eating their traditional diet.

We have made a gross error in calling cultures that have come before us "primitive." In the sense that they did not use or rely on complex, modern technology, this is correct. But the term is more often perceived as meaning "crude." In fact, these people were scientists; their laboratories were oceans, forests, their homes, and nature. They performed their tests on family, friends, animals, communities, and themselves. They had the same hunger as we do to discover how things work, and many of their discoveries were precursors to important advancements today—once dismissed as old wives' tales, only later to be confirmed by modern science.

Thus, Nature's Principle is based on science and nature according to many cultures that lived harmoniously and healthfully by harnessing and respecting nature, not by trying to reinvent or outsmart it. We are just beginning to understand this approach intellectually, yet many wise traditional cultures on the earth knew this intuitively and instinctually. Everyday statistics are proving that their approach to health and well-being was more effective than our current one. In our advanced cultures (if you exclude infant mortality rates), we are not living longer; we're dying longer.

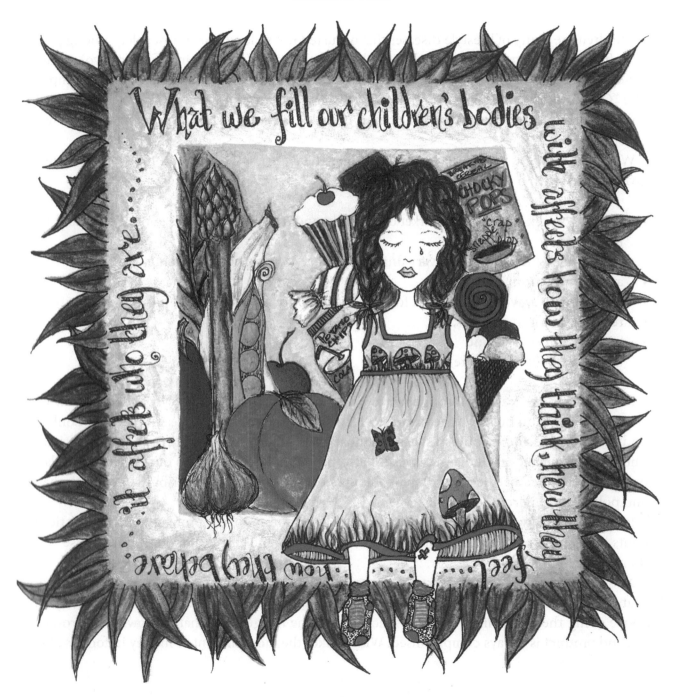

What we fill our children's bodies with affects how they think, how they feel... how they behave... it affects who they are.....

Children are dying of lifestyle diseases that occurred not so long ago almost solely among people over fifty. This concept is the antidote to the Lethal Recipe (covered in Chapter Two), which I believe creates the biggest danger we face as a species: self-annihilation through overconsumption. The "Consumption Concept" is a philosophy I share with you in detail in Chapter Four—and is a way to bring together everything I present in order to create a shift in thinking about how we consume.

What and how you eat impacts your whole life. The *Return to Food* philosophies are designed to give you the tools to learn how to:

- be able to walk into a supermarket confidently, and understand what is good for you and what is not;
- make the best decisions for every unique situation you find yourself facing;
- avoid temptation;
- learn how to crave and select the foods that will nourish, energize, and protect your body;
- reverse disease symptoms;
- have tons of energy; and
- create the body you desire and deserve.

I believe—as I've learned through my own life experiences and those of my clients—that what and how we eat and do life is the basis for everything. How and what we eat impacts not only our bodies and minds and emotional states and those who come in contact with us, but also our planet. The food that makes us lethargic and sick also produces litter that lines our streets and fills the oceans, and causes needless, exorbitant amounts of fossil fuels that contribute to climate change and pollute the environment.

Just as Wayne Dyer believes "there is a spiritual solution for every problem," many holistic students believe there is a natural solution for every ailment and that it first lies in the phrase "First, do no harm."

Nature's Principle is about observing nature. It is a guiding principle and not an absolute. I know that when it comes to food, when a management team, the CEO, or the shareholders place profits above doing the right thing, or ego is placed above the integrity of what is grown and produced, the end product is always compromised. What makes the most amount of money in food is always about cutting corners, systems, and speed. These are all rules that nature does not play by in food production. Nature has its own schedule, and when it follows this, there are more nutrients in the food without a negative impact on the planet, without the creation of chemicals, laboratories, and using animals to test it.

As part of nature, you don't need to diet; you simply need to follow the natural laws encoded in your DNA. When we tap into that knowledge, guided by our intuition, we access great universal truth. Science (as we know it) is just scraping the surface. We have much to learn and, when we combine this with an innate sense of what we should do, the results are powerful.

I've seen firsthand the power that this vital shift in mindset can have on people's relationship with food. It's not just hope for a better life but also immediate benefits that can cause positive change overnight. These changes then blossom into a lifetime of benefits.

Rather than telling others about a new diet, people become the change they wish to see in themselves and the world, the way Gandhi advised. They become who they dreamed they would be, who they are called to be. As a result, they inspire others to ask what it is they are doing or have done that has caused such amazing shifts in their lives.

This is the power of the philosophies that are based on Nature's Principle. The ripple effect is not only important but imperative; we are no longer thinking of generations alive today but also of those yet to come.

How we eat is a reflection of our mental, emotional, and spiritual state. Our choices with regard to our health and the state of our well-being are a reflection of the way we think. The philosophies and theories in this book are designed to provide a thought process that will enable you to develop your own critical thinking.

The anti-diet approach can be applied at any income and skill level, and will give you far more energy than it requires. It is not a quick fix but the way of lasting change; therefore, nothing you invest is a waste. This is not a fad, but a return to how things have worked best historically, not just for some but for all of us on this planet.

What is good for the planet is good for the people; what is truly good for the people is good for the planet.

Why waste a moment more? Act now, and the great thing is that in doing so you will add a dimension of quality to your life that will have you waking up, bouncing out of bed with amazing energy, a smile on your face, and your *ikigai* (a Japanese word meaning 'the reason for getting up in the morning') starting to build and get stronger.

CHAPTER TWO

THE LETHAL RECIPE

*"The general population doesn't know what's happening and it doesn't even
know it doesn't know."*
Noam Chomsky

WHEN "NATURAL" BECOMES "UNNATURAL"

When I first started publically speaking about nutrition, I told people all the horrible things
that were being done to our food. There was no internet yet, so most of my research was arduous and hard to find. There were no films like *Food, Inc.*, *Food Matters*, and *Fed Up*, or celebrity advocates warning us of the dangers of processed food.[1] I was so enraged by what was
happening that I overwhelmed audiences, and often they would leave my presentations
shell-shocked. Sadly, few of them made real changes—it's hard to take action when you're
overwhelmed. In addition, I had focused more on what was wrong with our food system than
on what they could do. I think it is important to be aware of what is wrong with our food
system, but at some point the accumulation of this information can be addictive and fatalistic.

*No matter how nutritionally powerful a food is, it can be turned into a toxic,
addictive substance with enough processing.*

The inconvenient truth, however, is that every single thing that is commoditized is vulnerable
to bastardization. If it's not organic, it probably contains GMOs (genetically modified organisms).
Most of the food on a typical supermarket shelf has been compromised in some way. There are ways
for you to get around this, and Chapters Three to Seven in this book provide solutions. You can go

directly to the solutions now, if you like. This chapter is simply about what has happened to most foods and why they are causing sickness. If I were to cover every food that's been altered, it would rival the expanse of information contained in Wikipedia. You don't need to know all this. You simply need to know how food is processed, how to identify processed food, and how to avoid it.

There's a common tip about food that suggests: if you can't pronounce it, you shouldn't be eating it. It's true, but it does not go far enough. There are many one-word ingredients on the super-market shelves that have been processed to the point of being addictive and toxic to the body.

Just because everything we eat comes initially from nature, does not mean by
the time we eat it, it is natural.

I define real food this way: if you can make it, create it, or produce it in your backyard or kitch-en with rudimentary materials (soaking nuts, sprouting seeds, drying and fermenting foods, for example), it is food. If it has come out of a laboratory or is the result of elaborate machinery and chemistry, it is not food. Margarine, artificial sweeteners, GMOs, and unpronounceable chemicals are obviously not foods. But beware: even in some organic foods, there are highly processed ingre-dients that are part of the Lethal Recipe.

Most people really don't take the time to even think about it. We eat what appeals to us from moment to moment. It's almost a no-brainer. We eat to satisfy cravings (without even thinking about where they're coming from); we eat to numb feelings and celebrate events; we eat and eat and eat … without too much thought or effort involved.

Society largely and blindly trusts the foods on the grocery store shelves. We trust the food manu-facturers, the government (US Food and Drug Administration [FDA], Canadian Food Inspection Agency, and other watchdog groups), our doctors, dietitians, and the marketers, many of whom have misled us with misinformation and food labels. In my many years of educating and public speaking, people would routinely become angry with me, saying that the government would just not allow what I'm telling them to be done to their food or to animals.

I'd love to think it's not the primary intention of big food companies to make food that will hurt us. But they are intentionally making food that makes them money, no matter how it impacts our health. Consumers play a part when they demand foods that are prepared faster, last longer, and cost less, and when we abdicate responsibility for knowing what is happening to our food, usually because we are too busy and consumed by other things to pay attention to, ask, demand, and be willing to pay for real food.

Most companies don't start out intending to make food that is deliberately bad for us. They don't think, "Let's make people really sick, deprive them of nutrients, add lots of dangerous toxins, and so on." They start out with the intention to make money and do so by producing products that sell. They solve what they perceive to be a problem—for example, kids don't like crusts on their bread, so they say, "Let's cut the crusts off." They say, "This single mom of three is too tired to cook after working all day, so let's make a meal she can throw in the microwave and eat in five minutes."

And although the intentions may not be lethal, lifestyle disease rates show that the results definitely are.

THE MAIN FIVE LETHAL RECIPE INGREDIENTS

Anything can become a Lethal Recipe ingredient with enough denaturing through heat, processing, removing nutrients, and exposure to toxic substances. This is what I refer to as the Lethal Recipe. There are five main ingredients in almost everything in the supermarket and it is the proliferation of these five ingredients in our diets that is, in the majority of cases, making us sick. Often, by simply removing them or returning to natural versions, you can reverse disease symptoms. The following five are not the only Lethal Recipe ingredients; there are many other foods that are processed the same way, such as dairy and soy.

- Refined oils
- Refined sugars
- Refined salts
- Refined grains
- Chemicals

Take out all of the products at the supermarket that contain one or more of these ingredients and almost nothing will be left on the shelves. You think I'm exaggerating? Conduct your own informal experiment and see for yourself.

Most of these ingredients started out in a natural state that was not harmful to us, but the extreme processing has changed their composition and turned them into lethal ingredients found in almost all of our commonly consumed grocery store foods.

The best way to explain this dangerous transformation from good to deadly is to use the example of the poppy flower. Poppy sap has natural opiates in them. If you remove the sap from the flower bud, dry it out, grind them into a powder (as they do in Iran), and consume this very natural substance, it will actually give you a feeling of well-being. It's not a highly addictive substance in its natural state, nor is it highly toxic to the body.

It's all in the processing. Extreme processing involves the use of high and intense heat, plus nutritional depletion (removal or destruction of macronutrients and micronutrients), plus the addition of chemicals. This combination equals sickness, addiction, and disease.

intense heat + nutritional depletion + chemicals = sickness, addiction, and disease

Processing the poppy sap removes macronutrients and micronutrients (such as fibres, vitamins, minerals, and phytonutrients, which are naturally occurring protective plant chemicals including compounds that create flavour, colour, and aroma) and changes the seeds' molecular structure, turning it into opium. The substance then becomes more addictive and toxic to the body. Processing it even further creates the pure substance known as heroin, highly addictive and detrimental to the body.

The process of how we create modern-day flours, oils, table salt, sugars, and chemicals is not dissimilar. When we eat food treated this way, minus the macro and micronutrients, our body says, "I am not getting what I want; feed me more." And because the macronutrients have been removed, making the food easier to chew and digest, you can actually eat more. In fact, if you take a food just even one step away from nature, by cooking it, you can eat more of that food.

Changing a food's structure, through synthetic fertilizers, chemical pesticide use, genetic modification, and processing, alters the effect the food would otherwise have on the body; less of the positive, more of the negative. The effect may show up overnight in the form of an allergy or it may take years to show up. Your genetic history and the way you live will determine the impact the food has. Every body is different.

As you can see, the exponential rise in disease directly corresponds with the processing of our foods and the introduction of the Lethal Recipe. We're overweight, yet often eating fat-free foods;

tired, yet unable to sleep; stressed and spending money on pills to help us cope—pills that only worsen the problem. But while we feel overwhelmed because we are stuck in this negative cycle, the solution to all of the problems, or at least most of these problems, is so simple—remove the Lethal Recipe from your Life Kitchen and return to food. The healthier and closer to nature we eat, the stronger, cleaner, and healthier our body will be. I notice that the better I eat, the clearer and more positive my thoughts are, and the less I am given to depression and negativity.

"Absence of proof of toxicity is not proof of safety."
Udo Erasmus

Start your shift to good health by listening to yourself. When you learn how a food is processed in such an extreme way (as described in the Oils section below), your common sense and intuition will tell you that it can't be good for you. There were people (regarded as extremists at the time) who protested oil processing when it began. They warned that it was unwise to consume these oils. In response, the scientific community, backed by the oil industry, asked, "Where is your proof?"

Well, to start with, the proof is in your gut, both literally and figuratively. But scientifically speaking, unfortunately, those using their common sense when this was first happening did not have the resources to amass the proof required to demonstrate the deleterious effects on the body. Now, more than thirty years later, we have proof of the toxic effects of processed and modified oils; it has been confirmed and is undeniable. Sadly, the oil industry has nevertheless distributed and sold the consumer on its product. It is almost impossible to eat a meal (unless you prepare it yourself) in which these bad oils do not exist. Over the years, we've been inundated with one-sided scientific misinformation that has the general public thinking that certain oils are not only harmless but good for the body. This couldn't be further from the truth. But because the effects of the Lethal Recipe are not always immediate—in the way that anaphylactic shock is—processed foods are often dismissed as a non-critical threat.

It is not my intention to scare you. Instead, I tell you these things to inform you, teach you to trust the signals your own body is giving you, and empower you to live a vibrant, healthy, and completely full life. Are you ready?

The Five Main Ingredients Globally Made With the Lethal Recipe

Oils

Oils were once rare and precious foods that—naturally made—were prone to spoiling after exposure to air, light, and heat. Today, oils are highly processed (to increase shelf life and thus increase profits) using such extreme procedures that their chemical bonds are changed and the way they affect DNA and our body are dramatically and dangerously altered.

Oils and fats are fundamental to our health. We need them in our diet for a good immune system, sharp brain function, cardiovascular health, and to provide us with energy. There are fats that nourish and protect the body against disease. But there are also fats that cause degenerative disease and can contribute, when eaten in excess over a long period of time, to death.

As soon as you cook or chemically refine oil, its nutritional benefits disappear and it becomes harmful. Most of the oils on the supermarket shelves are oils without nutritional benefits. In addition, exposure to air and light causes any fat to become rancid and toxic.

Check out the extreme processing your cooking oils go through before they reach you.

Eight Steps to Create Common Cooking Oil

Step 1: Cooking—the seeds or nuts are cooked, mashed, and then formed into a cake.
Step 2: Solvent extraction—hexane or heptane (gasoline) is combined with the cooked, mashed seed cake to remove the oil.
Step 3: Degumming—water and phosphoric acid remove phospholipids and many other nutrients.
Step 4: Refining—the oil is mixed with sodium hydroxide (caustic soda) and sometimes mixed with sodium carbonate.
Step 5: Bleaching—filters and acid-treated, activated clays are used to remove natural colours and aromas.
Step 6: Deodorizing—the above steps cause the oil to become distasteful and take on pungent

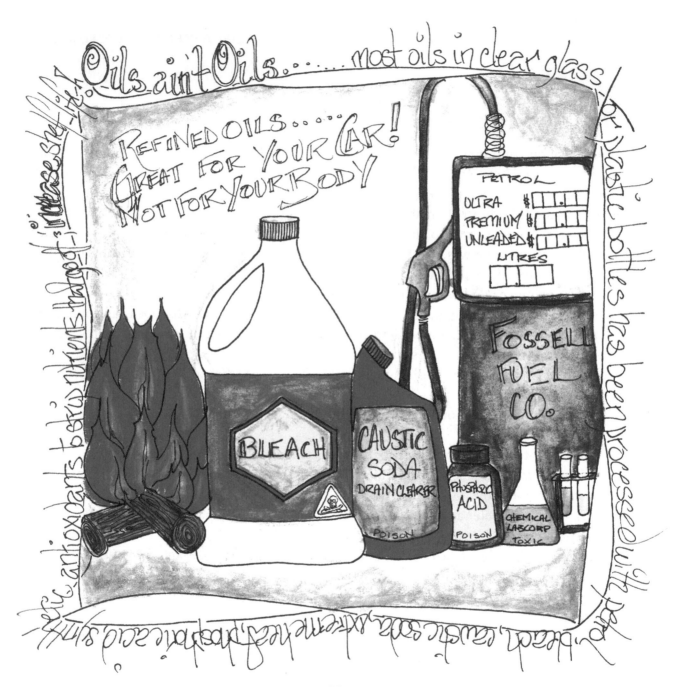

smells, which is not surprising. So it goes through another degenerating process of heating the oil to between 240° C and 270° C to render it tasteless and odourless. Plus, of course, now nutritionally useless and most likely harmful.

Step 7: Final preservation—most oils on the shelves of the supermarket are further treated to extend their shelf life. This can include the addition of synthetic antioxidants such as butylated hydroxytoluene, butylated hydroxyanisole, propyl gallate, tertiary butylhydroquinone, citric acid, and methyl silicone.

Step 8: A defoamer is then added before the final stage of bottling in a clear plastic bottle.

It doesn't take a team of scientists and dietitians to figure out that doing all this to a seed can render it harmful to consume. Hundreds of years ago, it wouldn't have taken a scientist to decide that a piece of rotting flesh was most likely not suitable to eat and possibly toxic. Today, unless you have a long list of research to verify your claim, gut instinct is considered the tool of a quack. But we were made with it for a reason. I strongly urge you to resist the pressure from the scientific and commercial community to distrust your instinct and intuition when questioning whether something is good or harmful for you.

If you require significant research to verify the information on fats, check out a fascinating and comprehensive book called *Fats that Heal, Fats that Kill* (1993) by internationally recognized expert on fats and oils, Udo Erasmus. It is illuminating.

For oils in my own kitchen I now choose only those that can be expressed naturally, without chemicals—like cold-pressed coconut oils, cold-pressed olive oil, and grass-fed butter—or by using rudimentary tools like stones. Any oils that cannot be made by hand are at the very least extracted with heptane and hexane, even flaxseed, chia seed, canola, sunflower, and soybean. I mainly use organic cold-pressed coconut oil and olive oil.

SUGAR

Sugar is the original sweetening ingredient in nature's desserts. Delicious, mouth-watering, pure, and, believe it or not, nutritious. You have to work hard to get sugar from its source or wait patiently for it to develop. You have to wait for fruit to ripen and then climb a tree. Honey and cane juices also require effort, risk, and caution. In their natural state, they all have naturally occurring protective

Sugar in nature is different to processed

REFINED **SUGAR**

as NATURAL

as HEROIN

'and' as GOOD FOR YOU TOO!

refined, genetically modified, chemically

treated nutrient-stripped sugars in most

kids who chew on fresh cane rarely get carious or diabetes

and never find them in the

processed foods today)

high fructose corn syrup is the crack cocaine of sugars, it isn't natural

sow in most

bees are dumped, fed refined sugar & corn meal as honey production

properties in the form of nutrients, and, perhaps because sugar is high in calories, nature makes us work for it.

The difference between the effects of refined sugar and natural cane sugar on the body was notably documented by Sir Frederick Banting, one of the first discoverers of insulin. His research in Panama in 1929 indicates that cane plantation owners who consumed large quantities of refined sugar commonly had diabetes, whereas plantation workers who had access only to the raw sugar cane to chew on had no incidence of diabetes. Research is now showing that many highly processed sugars and foods turn off the body's signal to stop eating and inhibit our desire to exercise.[2]

Refined or white sugar is not a natural product. Yes, it is obtained from a natural ingredient, but what is left after processing is a toxic and highly addictive substance. Here's a look at the process your table sugar goes through.

First, whole cane juice is clarified using heat and lime (calcium hydroxide, not the fruit). It is boiled down, crystallized, and placed it in a centrifuge to remove the molasses. The sucrose crystals are dissolved and the sugar is then decolourized, using granular carbon to absorb the unwanted molecules. What's left is 99.8 percent pure sucrose, devoid of any nutritionally redeemable qualities. In its refined state, sugar has absolutely no protective properties.

Sugar cane, when it is simply juiced and dehydrated, is brown with textured bits in it; it has a lovely, gentle flavour. You can get powdered versions like coconut palm sugar or dehydrated cane juice in reputable health-food stores or organic grocers. It will cost you around seven to ten dollars for about a pound, and it still contains naturally present minerals and vitamins.

The World's Biggest Socially Acceptable, Cheap Addiction

Never underestimate the addictive power of sugar. It can take years to break the habit and be harder than heroin or cocaine to break free from. In addition, it's the cheapest "drug" on earth, found everywhere and socially acceptable. We're rewarded with it, even. It's no joke, this sugar addiction.

Sugar is linked to over 178 diseases and illnesses! It is a major contributor to malnutrition in overfed nations, as it strips nutrients from the body and unbalances your entire body chemistry. Westerners are eating on average 150 pounds a year of the white stuff.

Some of the major conditions that are directly attributed to the consumption of sugar are osteoporosis (due to calcium leaching to balance the acidity of sugar), diabetes, depression, anxiety,

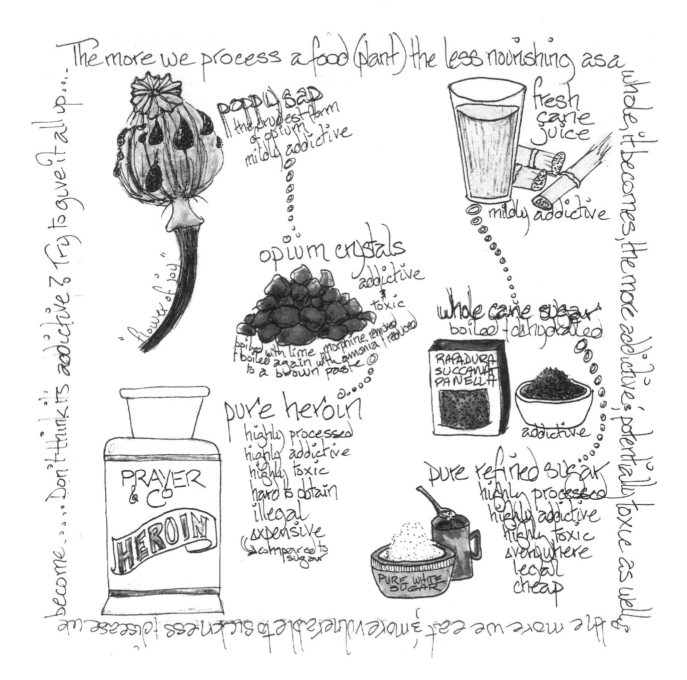

The more we process a food (plant) the less nourishing as a whole it becomes, the more addictive, potentially toxic as well...

poppy sap
the purest form
of opium
mildly addictive

"flower of joy"

opium crystals
addictive
+ toxic
boiled with lime morphine removed
+ boiled again with amonia reduced
to a brown paste

pure heroin
highly processed
highly addictive
highly toxic
hard to obtain
illegal
expensive
(compared to sugar)

PRAYER & CO
HEROIN

fresh cane juice
mildly addictive

whole cane sugar
boiled + dehydrated
RAPADURA
SUCCANAT
PANELLA
addictive

pure refined sugar
highly processed
highly addictive
highly toxic
everywhere
legal
cheap

PURE WHITE SUGAR

Don't think it's addictive? Try to give it all up...

become...the more we eat; more vulnerable to sickness + disease we

29

heartburn, and cancer. Dr. Nancy Appleton lists over 140 ways sugar can ruin your health in her books *Lick the Sugar Habit* (2002) and *Suicide by Sugar* (2008). As early as 1931, Nobel Prize winner Dr. Otto Warburg discovered that cancer feeds on sugar.

After eating refined sugar, observe the effect it has on your ability to think clearly and maintain level moods. Many people notice depression, anxiety, headaches, or brain fog. Most people have observed hyperactivity in children after a sugar hit, a reaction that often turns into tears, anger, or frustration.

Refined sugar can also trigger a desire to eat more even though we're not hungry. It can trigger a compulsion to eat something salty to balance out the flavour of an extreme sugar hit or to eat protein, as your body's way of balancing your blood sugar.[3]

High Fructose Corn Syrup

As I've noted, highly processed foods have been shown to shut off the mechanism that signals our bodies that we've had enough. I also mentioned that since highly processed foods lack nutrients, the body signals us to eat more because it's not getting what it needs. So we unknowingly eat more of the wrong foods, adding empty calories bite by bite, but not the nutrients our bodies desperately crave.

And when you eat refined sugars, particularly high fructose corn syrup, the problems with nutrient deficiency pile up even faster. It's been found that when the body is attempting to digest high fructose corn syrup, it actually has to use stored-up nutrients to do so. You're not only getting virtually no nutrients when you eat, you're actually losing nutrients. So the "empty calories" are really robbing nutrients from your body, while causing you to overeat.

Don't forget that weight gain is only one of the problems these foods cause. As I've noted, processed foods, including refined sugars, have been linked to every lifestyle disease imaginable, including autism, Multiple Sclerosis, and liver damage.

Artificial Sweeteners

Artificial sweeteners are even further away from nature than white table sugar; they could never be made in nature. Even ones that say they are sourced from natural ingredients (like xylitol and

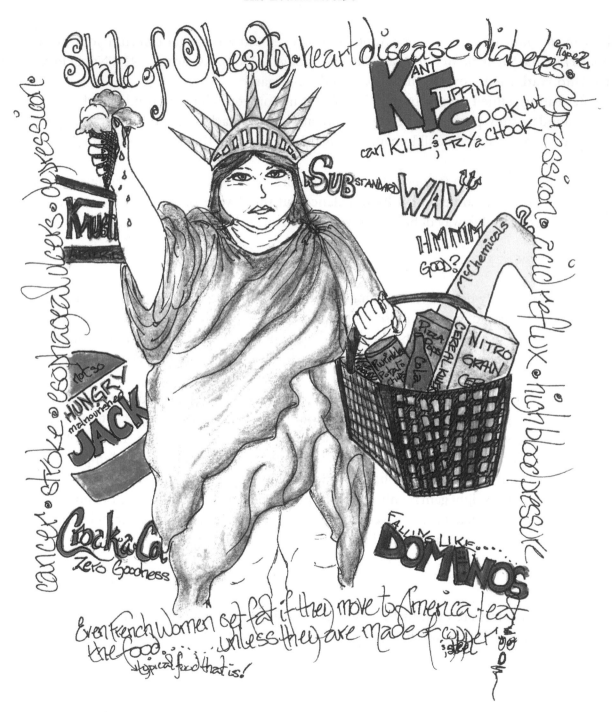

white stevia) are in fact highly processed and foreign to the body. Artificial sweetners are classified as excitotoxins, which are neurotoxins known to contribute to many brain disorders: they stimulate the neurons in the brain to such an extreme point that they actually die.

The FDA has logged ninety-two side effects from the consumption of excitotoxins. Here is an honest look at just a few of the conditions linked to their consumption.

- Brain damage
- Neurological disorders associated with seizures
- Disorders of the endocrine system
- Obesity
- Infections
- Abnormal development of the nervous system
- Links to effects on the development of diseases such as Alzheimer's, Parkinson's, ALS, MS, and Huntington's disease.

Excitotoxins are in virtually every type of food product you can think of. They go by the names aspartame (found in NutraSweet, Splenda, Xylitol, and Equal), MSG, and hydrolyzed vegetable proteins. They're not just bad for your health—they are addictive. I've had clients who broke free of their alcohol addiction but were unable to drop the addictive products in their diet, which always contained excitotoxins—that's what kept them hooked.

The premise of these artificial sweeteners is that you'll lose weight, but I've discovered through research and my practical work that the very opposite is true. I have many clients who—by making no other changes than removing artificial sweeteners from their diets—have finally lost weight. One client, Jeremy, lost twenty-four pounds in one month by replacing his Coke Zero habit with spring water.

When the toxins are removed, in this case artificial sweeteners and excitotoxins, the body stops creating fat cells to store them. You lose weight, your health improves, and you experience a huge increase in the quality of your life.

Replace the White Stuff with the Right Stuff

We are led to believe that if we don't eat three meals a day, every day, 365 days a year, we are going to suffer from malnutrition. The fact is, we don't require a large volume of nutrient-rich food for vibrant health. It is a matter of removing artificial sweeteners from your diet. Choose sweeteners that are close to nature: good options are raw, unpasteurized honey; dried fruits; coconut palm sugar; and dehydrated cane juice.

Salt

Salt in its natural state can have eighty-four-plus minerals in it. That's just what we know of at this time. Today, most, if not all, the minerals are gone, except sodium chloride, and other additives (that the consumer doesn't get to know about), which are put back into salt. Most table salts contain up to seven different ingredients, including sugar and anticaking agents. Some of these are inorganic and insoluble ingredients. The only one that is disclosed is the anticaking agent, which is chalk.

Table salts are heated to extremely high temperatures—almost 800° C or 1,500° F—to bind them together. Then they are ground. Today, salt is a refined food that is not only easy to obtain but also difficult to avoid, unless you cook your own food from scratch.

Salt is vital for our health, but little is needed for most people to maintain good health. It is a great flavour enhancer, but too much can mask and take away from the beauty of natural-food flavours. As a chef, I can tell you that table salt tastes bitter, metallic, and acrid, and those flavours are imparted to the foods you cook. Although subtle, table salt's flavour is very distinct to a sensitive and discriminating palate.

Seventy percent of our salt consumption comes from processed foods, so the very best way to lower your salt intake is limit your processed-food consumption; cook at home from scratch. It is easy, then, to avoid over salting, as the taste alone will repel you, unlike "hidden salts" that are almost tasteless yet highly addictive.

Salts in processed foods are referred to as "hidden salts" because we are not aware of them—they don't always taste overtly salty. Read the labels and you will find out some pretty amazing facts about the foods you choose. Some breakfast cereals can have the equivalent of one teaspoon of sodium per serving and not even taste salty.

Replacing your table salt with a natural sea salt that is hand harvested and doesn't have any additives, including anticaking agents, is the best way to start.

GRAINS

Non-cultivated grains were once highly nutritious in their sprouted or green form, only they are much better suited as food to large mammals who have mandibles and guts that can chew and digest grains in their raw form. The grain we eat today is a highly processed version that has been hybridized and scientifically manipulated to grow in specific conditions to create a more desirable result in food manufacturing. Treated grains have a dramatically different effect on the body than a whole, raw, organic, wild grain would.

Whole grains today are not just modified but also sprayed with chemical pesticides from the time they are seeds to when they are fully grown. They are sprayed with synthetic fertilizers, grown in soil that does not regenerate naturally, and stored for months where they can develop mycotoxins and aflatoxins, which remove any life-giving nutrients that may be left.

Refined grains are modified by removing the bran and the germ, and then ground at high speeds, which creates heat that denatures the proteins and changes their structure. The result is processed further through grinding and sifting. The whole grains can then be sprayed in storage, gassed, and combined with corrosive bleaching chemicals to achieve white flour. In our gut, this form of white flour forms a glue like substance that looks like toothpaste and is more like a loose bread dough before baking. This gut glue can actually mow down the microscopic, beneficial villi in the gut, thus inhibiting nutrient absorption and creating all kinds of gut issues and disorders.

In my kitchen, I have organic sprouted spelt kernels, which I mill in my high-powered blender when I want flour. You can do this with grains and some seeds, like quinoa, for an alternative to processed flours. Remember to find organic versions if you want the flours ground beforehand.

CHEMICALS

There are tens of thousands of chemicals in our foods today, from pesticide residue to that of chemicals used in processing, and from hidden ones used in nanotechnology to those deliberately added to our food. Most have not been tested adequately for safety; even fewer have been tested for safety in children; and virtually none have been tested in the chemical cocktail combinations that are found in in our food.

It would be almost impossible to have such a task completed, as the time and resources to do all of this properly would be enormous, and with no money to be made from it, the chances of it happening are slim to none. One of the main purposes of this book (and my seminars) is to teach you, urge you, not to wait for scientific studies to convince you to make changes. If you wait, your body could be riddled with disease and pain before one such study has emerged. The truth remains the truth even in the absence of scientific data.

The chemicals we ingest do not just go through our bowels and out the trap door. They can permeate every cell of our body, as shown by the presence of chemicals and pesticide residue found in breast milk and the placenta. We can store them for years. In fact, we have found now that when buried, the human body does not break down and decompose as it once did.

Preserving, as one might with formaldehyde, does not prolong life; it merely prevents the powerful natural inclination of dead things to decompose. Most people wouldn't dream of eating a piece of meat preserved with formaldehyde, yet we eat food infused with preservatives just as powerful.

DAIRY AND MAMMOTH MOO-MYTHS

Nothing in my work educating people about food brings up as many emotional responses as the thought of not being able to drink milk and eat dairy. The questions I'm asked most by audiences are about milk. "Do I really need as much as they say? The choices are endless: what are the best milks to drink? How much butter, cheese, and yogurt do I need? Should I be eating these foods at all? Organic, low-fat, skim, calcium-enriched? Help!"

Perhaps this anxiety and fear is caused by our intuitive connection with milk, because of our mothers, and how, if we were breastfed, it sustained us early on. Despite the fact that our mothers are not cows and we are not calves, somehow there has been a transference of our desire for milk and milk products to a prevalent belief that we need cows' milk to survive and be healthy beyond weaning. Ironically, like all mammals (including humans), not even cows need milk beyond weaning.

The story of milk shares a similar theme to the other staples of the Lethal Recipe—that is, sugar, salt, oils/fats, grains, and chemicals. When you take milk out of its natural context, with respect to how you treat it, consumption increases, quality decreases, and sickness is born.

Milk is a powerful multibillion-dollar global industry, and there is a massive machine set up to protect its interests and promote dairy consumption. Independent research on the benefits of dairy is rare. Advertising is clever, and to endorse products, they use credible, trusted experts, often in the form of doctors (who only study nutrition six to seven weeks at the most during their twelve years of medicine) giving nutritional advice.

There is no question about it: milk is an amazing food—no matter what animal it comes from—for young creatures after they're born. But all mammals are designed to wean off milk. Their body creates intolerance to milk and stops producing the enzymes to break down its nutrients; this is the natural incentive to wean off milk. As with all things in nature, we are just beginning to understand it. It is life-giving only to the offspring it is designed for.

In its most natural state—that is, raw—milk is most beneficial for calves. Keep in mind that a cow's milk is designed to help grow a calf to hundreds of pounds in size. Pasteurization activists are so extreme in their positions that I wonder when they will suggest legislation requiring human mother's milk to be pasteurized. Absurd perhaps, but it comes to the root of the issue. You wouldn't think of pasteurizing milk to give to an animal's offspring, because it is so fresh and close to the source.

When you buy dairy products, you participate in the practice of day-old calves being removed from their mothers, as the cow will not produce milk on the scale that "big dairy" demands with the calf still feeding from her. So we, not the naturally intended offspring for the milk, consume it instead. As milk became a big business to feed the masses, not only were we drinking it far from the source, but it also came from thousands of beasts, and if one was sick, it wasn't one calf that risked its life but thousands of people who were potentially put at risk.

Louis Pasteur discovered that if you cook milk to a certain point, many of the potentially harmful bacteria are killed off; cook it too much, though, and it tastes disgusting. So in the name of potentially saving thousands, milk is now cooked and, in the process, is rendered devoid of much, if not most, of the good bacteria.

Our milk on the shelves is not just pasteurized—it is homogenized, clarified, and can undergo many processes that take it from natural to unnatural. These extreme processes could never be replicated in nature. Such milk is now being linked with many lifestyle illnesses. When milk undergoes these extreme processing procedures, it no longer has an alkalinizing effect on the body; instead, it becomes acidic. It is a known and proven fact that disease becomes active and is fostered in overly acidic bodies.

I've seen hundreds of people over the years remove all kinds of health issues by removing pasteurized dairy from their diet.

See www.returntofood.com/dairy for the ten most commonly asked questions about milk.

ANDREW

Many people go to their doctors to get their illnesses diagnosed. The medical system's ability to diagnose and surgically treat disease is impressive. But most doctors are not professionally educated on holistic nutrition and its ability to heal. There is a growing trend of high-profile doctors using food as part of their tool kit, but they are the exception, not the rule, and the disparity in their knowledge is great.

I spoke at the beginning of this book about Andrew, who came to me newly diagnosed with Type 2 Diabetes. He had his prescription in hand as well as the diet the doctor had suggested. Looking at the diet, I began to cross out the foods that I knew were not healing; some were actually part of the Lethal Recipe. By the time I got to the bottom of the list, it was almost entirely crossed out. "Andrew," I said, "this diet looks like it was prepared by a drug company. It seems like it's designed to lower your blood sugar, but it also provides enough foods to keep you dependent on insulin. And there's nothing on the list that would actually heal your pancreas." The pancreas is vital in the production of insulin to lower blood sugar; it can become overtaxed when we eat too much sugar over a sustained period of time. Soon, it wears out and cannot keep up with the body's demand for insulin. The health of the pancreas can be restored by removing sugars and eating living, healing foods.

I looked down at the fine print at the bottom of the page listing the recommended foods, and it was in fact prescribed by the pharmaceutical company of the exact drug Andrew had in his hand.

Within seven days of working together to eliminate the Lethal Recipe from his diet, HyperNourishing him, and having him eat primarily plant foods, all of Andrew's diabetic symptoms disappeared, and while he was following my guidelines, he did not need insulin.

IF YOU'RE GOING TO EAT MEAT

You eat whatever you eat eats.

Eating meat isn't a requirement for human survival.[4] Millions of vegetarians are testament to this, and I've met some incredibly fit and healthy vegans and vegetarians. Contrary to what some may believe, non-meat eaters are not all pale, wispy-thin people who are unable to hold their heads up due to weakness. I've met unhealthy vegetarians who eat a highly processed diet that would make any meat eater weak and pale, but I've met more unhealthy carnivorous people. You can be malnourished and unhealthy no matter what kind of dietary preference you have if your diet is unnatural and highly processed. The key to health is in how you eat, the quality of what you eat, and how natural it is.

People ask me all the time, "Should I stop eating meat?" I tell them that if they're going to eat meat, they would be wise to do so according to Nature's Principle and the Consumption Concept (described in Chapters Three and Four), and according to their own conscience. But it's also important to get educated, because how we are eating meat is completely unsustainable for the globe and its population.

Think about what you'd actually be willing to kill and in what order. Would you find it easier to kill a chicken or a fish? Most people say fish. And you know that fish tends to be healthier for us than chicken. Then move it up to the next level. Would you choose to kill a chicken or a lamb? A chicken or a cow?

The point here is this: we are less likely to want to kill that which is less healthy for us. This is an interesting truth I've observed in most omnivores. When we're unfettered by imbalance, our bodies and minds naturally give us the inclination to eat what is best for us. We simply need to reconnect with our natural state and listen to it.

A funny thing happens when we have to source our food from nature: we often choose the opposite of what we would in the processed world, where things are done for us. The reason is simple—we have stronger physiological impulses for things that are hard to obtain in nature. In nature, back when we had to find our food, this ensured we got enough but also controlled our portions. Also, we expended a great deal of exertion, which in the process strengthened and cleansed our body.

Based on consumption figures of restaurants in Western countries, given a choice between fish and chicken, most people choose chicken; between chicken and lamb, the choice is lamb; and between lamb and beef, more people choose beef.

Given the same choices, except that you have to kill, skin, bleed, gut, and prepare your meat, most people would choose lamb over beef, chicken over lamb, and fish over chicken. It seems that the less we identify with a beast, the easier it is to kill it.

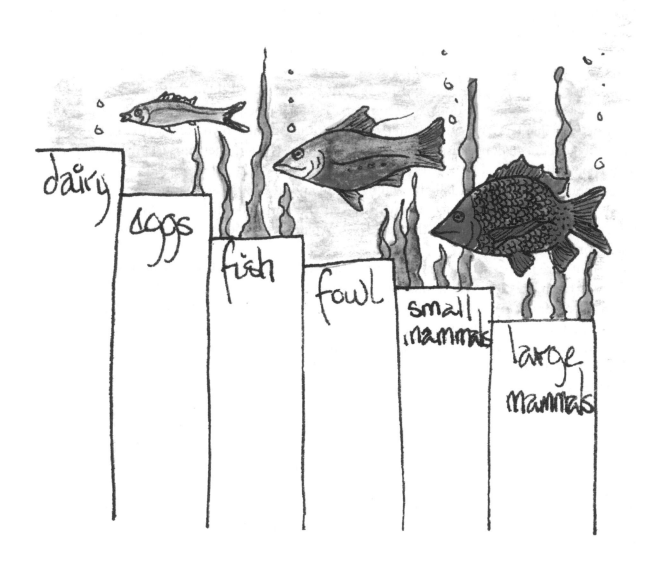

If you are going to eat animals, please consider the following. Any form of animal or fish protein requires ten to three hundred times the water of any plant protein to procure. There are many substances coursing through the body of an animal. The larger the animal, even an animal fed an organic diet, the more impact these substances have on the human body. My observation is that meat is addictive, and what we often mistake as a surge of well-being is actually a surge of the hormones and drugs from the animal's body.

The health of animal protein is a direct reflection on how well—humanely or inhumanely—the animal was raised, housed, fed, cared for, and butchered. Joel Salatin of Polyface Farms, the farmer featured in the *Food, Inc.* documentary, says an animal should have only one bad day in its life—the day it dies. If you are going to eat meat, choose that meat wisely, as how it lives and dies affects you and the environment. What it eats, you eat, and the more meat you eat, the greater the footprint you have on this planet.

Farmed fish is not a natural or environmentally sound alternative to eating seafood. It is true that we have fished many species to extinction and upset the balance of the oceans. The key is to figure out how to bring wisdom into the solution, not create more problems, as evidenced in fish farming that pollutes the water and is creating disease that can threaten wild species. "OceanWise" programs are a great start to selecting fish to eat, but also consider sustainably harvested sea vegetables, which can provide many fabulous nutrients.

I mentioned earlier that consuming meat isn't necessary for survival. But nor is it necessary for protein. Most people, when they encounter vegans or vegetarians, first wonder how they get their protein. In fact, meat or flesh protein isn't the best source of protein for the body, just as dairy isn't the best source of calcium for the human body. This has to do with how we metabolize the protein or calcium but also with the state of the animal from which the protein comes.

The typical meats sold in a grocery store often are from unhealthy, unhappy, very sick animals. The treatment of the animals determines the quality of the meat, which in turn affects your own health. Feedlots, caged-chicken farming systems, and pretty much any large-scale meat production will use practices that are not only unnatural but barbaric. Force-feeding, regular courses of antibiotics whether or not the animal is ill, steroid and hormone injections…these are just a few of the practices you can come across. The feed given to most of these animals is so far from their natural diets, it creates unhealthy animals, just like what happens to us when we eat foods that are unnatural for us. Typical feedlots give grain to cattle, even though their natural diet is grass. The grain causes bloating and in some cases death. I've seen footage of a hole being punctured into the side of a cow simply to relieve the malaise that comes from the gas and bloating. In extreme cases, some commercial feedlots feed stale candy to cattle to reduce costs, sometimes even candy still in their wrappers.

Meat from cattle raised on grass and legumes is five times higher in conjugated linoleic acid (CLA), which has been said to guard against cancer, heart disease, kidney disease, and obesity, than meat from feedlot cattle. It is also higher in vitamin E, beta carotene, and omega-3 fatty acids. And that difference is just from how they eat. What about how they're treated? While I'm not a vegetarian or an animal liberationist, I do believe animals deserve a decent life—even more so if they are being sacrificed for food. At the very least, could we not do this as traditional cultures did, giving reverence to a life that was given so we may eat?

Aside from the ethical and dietary factors, though, the truth is that if you eat animals that are mistreated, your body will get the end results of that ill treated meat—because it will be filled with stress and fear hormones, at the very least. It's just like when a baby breastfeeds. If the mother consumes alcohol or does drugs or eats badly, whatever she consumes is passed to her infant. Likewise, as we know, how she feels affects what is passed to her child.

If you want to know more about how food animals are treated and what's happening to your meat before it reaches the grocery shelves, start by reading Jeremy Rifkin's book, *Beyond Beef* (1992). Caution: I would read this book with a box of tissues nearby.

LOW-FAT, NONFAT FOODS

> *Is it a coincidence that the countries with the most low-fat, no-fat, fake-fat,*
> *low-sugar, no-sugar, fake-sugar food consumption are the countries with the*
> *highest incidence of heart disease, diabetes, cancers, and obesity rates?*

Many of the ingredients in low-fat and nonfat products are synthetic and create a toxic environment in the body while offering little to no nutrition.

Olestra—as an example—was created by Procter & Gamble to increase premature babies' intake of fat. Olestra is formed from sucrose (table sugar), and its fat molecules are so large and dense that it's impossible for the body to absorb or digest them. It also binds to vitamins and minerals, preventing their digestion.

In 1987, Procter & Gamble petitioned the FDA to approve Olestra as a general fat substitute. Coincidently, a stock analyst (Hercules Segalas) predicted that Olestra would be the biggest moneymaker in Procter & Gamble's history, generating upwards of $1.5 billion in annual sales. For nine years, Procter & Gamble lobbied and spent millions of dollars on their campaign, and in 1996, the FDA approved Olestra for use in "savoury snacks," as long as it had the following warning: "This product contains Olestra. Olestra may cause abdominal cramping and loose stools. Olestra inhibits the absorption of some vitamins and other nutrients. Vitamins A, D, E, and K have been added."

The warning has since been removed from packaging.

Now consider something from nature—organic broccoli, for example. No money was spent to convince the FDA it's safe for consumption.

Food tastes good because of the natural fats and flavor compounds found in it. When you process to remove fat, or naturally occurring sugars, you also lose taste. Thus, chemicals and synthetic ingredients, as well as colours, are added to make the food flavourful and appealing. These ingredients—think of the Lethal Recipe—are often addictive. As I mentioned before, when our food is devoid of the natural nutrients we need, we crave more, usually processed food, instead of fruits or vegetables, for example. The chemicals we eat create imbalance, and that imbalance causes us to desire the wrong foods and ultimately become unhealthy. In addition, when people consume low-fat or nonfat food, they often feel as though they're allowed to eat more because it's low-fat or fat-free. Do you see where this is heading?

When you start eating according to Nature's Principle and choosing fresh, whole foods, you'll eat less processed food. When you give your body the nutrients it needs, the cravings begin to diminish.

Flavourings and Colourings

Many of the ingredients found in flavourings and colourings just can't be found in nature—that should be your first red flag.

Some "flavourings" have as many as *four hundred* ingredients, and the companies making them aren't required to list these ingredients, since the product is patent protected. That means you don't really know what you're putting in your body at all.

Food colours and dyes are also a threat to our health—to begin with, they're either synthetic or chemically produced. Even colours derived from natural foods can cause health issues; they are extracted by solvents, like acetone, that can also remain in the colour after processing.

We are attracted to the various colours of real foods for certain reasons, usually depending on what they contain and what we need. Many of us still feel that instinctual pull to eat only food that is in season, for the same reason, thereby also avoiding foods that have been induced to grow outside their natural time. These foods do not taste nearly as vibrant as the ones grown naturally when they're supposed to, nor do they contain the same levels of nutrients. The body and mind, when working as nature intended, work together to guide us to healthy eating choices.

But what happens when these natural, colourful foods are processed? You got it: just as I said above, they lose their colours and nutrients. Even real food loses its colour and nutrients when all we do is blend it. Take the bountiful blueberry for example. Picked ripe, it is a deep, dark purple colour, and very rich in phytonutrients. The colour is so intense, it can actually stain your fingers and mouth. Now, put those blueberries into a blender. Once blended, the mixture is purple, but a lighter purple than it first was. Leave it out for just five minutes and the colour lightens even more as the drink oxidizes. Through oxidation, nutrients are being lost. If this mixture sits for a few hours, it becomes almost greyish in colour.

Natural colour allows us to tell whether or not a food is fresh. When you consider highly processed foods, which are definitely not fresh, you can imagine that most of them are a very dull, ugly colour we would not be drawn to and would in fact avoid. In addition, they are rendered virtually tasteless. The clever food manufacturers know this, so they add dyes and flavours to ensure our attraction to their foods. Our instincts are tricked and most of us are never even aware this is happening.

To make matters worse, the artificial and added flavours are addictive. Think about potato chips and candy. The salt, sugar, and intense flavouring prevents us from eating these foods in moderation. Remember the slogan "Bet you can't eat just one?" Of course the potato chip company says that. They know the effects of their ingredients—and we certainly end up eating more, just as we do because our food is nutrient-deficient.

There are literally thousands of chemicals combined in our foods from colours and flavourings. Many of these ingredients haven't even been tested for safety for consumption by children.[5] If you're living according to Nature's Principle, however, you won't wait for a study to tell you what to eat and what to avoid. One way to tell if your body is suffering from these dangerous additives is to cut them out of your diet for thirty days and see if you notice a difference.

THE DRUG-LIKE EFFECTS OF NATURAL FOOD VS PROCESSED FOOD

Certain foods can create a drug-like effect on our bodies. Even natural foods. Chocolate contains theobromine, a stimulant that works with caffeine, also in chocolate, to produce a "high"; sugar gives us a "rush" because of elevated glucose levels in our bloodstream (but beware the inevitable "crash" that will soon follow because of the resulting insulin release!); and tryptophan (found in protein-based foods including but not exclusive to meats, chocolate, oats, egg whites, dried dates, dairy, fish, poultry, sunflower, and sesame seeds) triggers serotonin production, which promotes feelings of safety and well-being.

Found in their most natural state, these foods and their natural chemicals are not harmful. However, when these same foods are highly processed, the naturally-occurring chemicals—that once produced subtle effects—now become like hard drugs. You get the same effect, only drastically intensified. Likewise, the corresponding low (after the initial high) is much lower than when you eat the food in its natural state. The body then naturally craves the high again (especially with a very low state of "low"), so we consume more of that food or another food that produces that same drug-like state of being. This creates a cycle of eating based on how the food makes us feel. We become addicted to the feelings—just like an alcoholic or drug addict—and we can't stop the cycle; it's just too painful.

Often, we don't even realize what's going on or that our food is the culprit. Remember the example of the poppy sap? Once we apply extreme processing to something, it can transform from a natural, harmless chemical to an extremely dangerous, addictive one—in the case of poppy sap, heroin. This is happening with processed foods every day.

NOURISH YOUR WAY OUT OF ADDICTION

In a study on the effects of nutrition on food choice, when malnourished lab rats were given a choice between alcohol and water, they always chose the alcohol. When their diets were supplemented with proper nutrition, they consistently chose the water over the alcohol. When returned to a nutrient-deficient diet—equivalent to our SAD (Standard American Diet)—they once again chose the alcohol over the water.[6]

Poor nutrition breeds poor food choices and consistently results in behavioural problems. I've observed amazing transformations time and time again, including the disappearance of cravings for addictive substances and activities, when people replaced the Lethal Recipe with *Return to Food*.

When giving up or trying to reduce cravings for addictive substances, the best thing you can do is build a healthy gut environment and immune system. Because it's involved in so many bodily processes, a healthy gut is the crux of our well-being. Poor gut health depresses our immune system and negatively affects our nervous system as well. It can cause all sorts of gastrointestinal issues but also ailments such as yeast infections, brain fog, anxiety, depression, and addiction through cravings.

The first step to creating a healthy gut is to remove all the toxins that could be causing it stress, such as processed foods, alcohol, sugar, bad fats, and caffeine. You can nourish your gut instead with a wide variety of minimally processed whole plant foods. As a result, the physiological side to the compulsive cravings will diminish, because your body is getting what it needs.

Nature is always seeking balance. Non-toxic foods in their whole, raw state and obtained based on bioavailability always deliver balance and do not send the body into extreme highs and lows. Nature also has an inherent protective mechanism for halting addiction. Most substances in their natural state aren't highly addictive and, if they are, nature makes them more difficult to obtain. Coffee is first fermented and roasted before we get addicted to it. Fermented black tea is more addictive than the naturally dried unfermented green tea. When you consider it takes about ten pounds of milk to create one pound of cheese, it makes sense that cheese contains more concentrated levels of addictive casomorphins and opioids than milk. Think, too, of wine versus grape juice. Tobacco and marijuana are dried or treated before they are turned into highly addictive substances.

In nature, we have to work harder to get sugars, fats, and proteins. It's smart! How much honey would you eat if you had to source it? How many nuts or seeds would you eat in a sitting if you had to climb the tree or harvest plants, and then break open the tricky layers that reveal the enzyme-rich raw seed or nut? How many and which animals would you eat if you had to kill and then process—bleed, gut, skin/pluck, disembowel—them yourself? Nature helps keep us from overindulging, which also ensures sustainability.

TIM

A client I had many years ago was an alcoholic who was aware he was drinking himself to death. He flew me out from Australia to do a lifestyle makeover and showed up so drunk at the airport to collect me, that he could hardly speak.

Within two weeks of my detoxing and HyperNourishing him, he no longer craved the alcohol. He actually found it harder to wean himself off diet drinks. Today, seven years later, Tim is alive, sixty pounds lighter, and sober.

GMOs: Genetically Modified Organisms

The term "GMO," or "genetically modified organism," refers to a plant, animal, or micro-organism whose gene structure has been altered in order to give it characteristics it doesn't naturally possess.

Take, for example, the tomato. It's a delicious, highly nutritious food. Eaten locally and in season, it provides a plethora of healthy nutrients. But consumers want to eat tomatoes year round, so scientists found a way to meet this demand. When you insert a fish gene into the tomato, the once warm-weather, summer food can be grown year-round. Convenient? Yes. Healthy? Well, that remains to be seen. But again we go back to what this book is all about—trusting yourself and nature in knowing what to eat and what to avoid. You don't have to wait for scientific studies and data to tell you how to eat. It's intuitive if you are ready to listen again.

Soybeans and corn are the two most genetically modified crops. Cotton, canola oil (rapeseed), and potatoes are the next most common GM products. Farmers have widely adopted GM technology: "Between 1996 and 2011, the total surface area of land cultivated with GM crops had increased by a factor of 94, from 17,000 square kilometers (4,200,000 acres) to 1,600,000 km² (395 million acres). 10% of the world's crop lands were planted with GM crops in 2010. As of 2011, 11 different transgenic crops were grown commercially on 395 million acres (160 million hectares) in 29 countries.[7]"

Another example of a GMO in our diets is the recombinant Bovine Growth Hormone (rBVG) in milk. This is a genetically engineered growth hormone that is injected into dairy cows to increase their milk production by 10 to 15 percent. Although its use is banned in Europe and Canada, boycotted by 95 percent of US farmers, and the US General Accountability Office and Consumers Union have issued warnings about its hazards for human health, the FDA still approves its usage.

Thanks to industry pressure, products derived from milk with rBVG aren't labelled as such and consumers have no way of identifying these potentially dangerous products. There are only certain products that are labelled as GMO-free products.

And what about the cows themselves? rBVG is like "crack for cows." It revs them up and makes them sick. Studies show that cows injected with rBVG have an increased chance of certain illnesses, a claim even the FDA admits.

The impact of these foods on the human body is not fully known and the companies who produce them do not want you to know what foods they are contained in.[8] Fine: when you are following your instincts and eating according to Nature's Principle, you will most certainly avoid any GMO, simply because it's not natural.

In his book *Seeds of Deception* (2003), Jeffrey M. Smith, executive director of the Institute of Responsible Technology, writes about different animals that are given the choice to eat either conventional seed or GM seed. Whether they are in the wild or in captivity, these animals always choose the conventional seed. They eat the GM seed only as a last resort. They know instinctively to avoid the altered food—an instinct many of us are missing. But we can follow their lead and our own instincts and choose real food—the way nature gives it to us.

Once you research Monsanto and what it has done globally with dangerous and even lethal chemicals (like Agent Orange, DDT, PCBs, and Saccharin), and how they've been linked to hundreds of thousands of farmers in India committing suicide, it is incredibly difficult to hold the space for love and forgiveness. I don't say this lightly: what companies like Monsanto are doing to farmers and our food globally is reprehensible and evil. Seventy to 80 percent of the food system has GMOs in it, and unless you are eating organic, you can be pretty much assured that there are GMOs in your food.

If you want to know more about GMOs, read *Genetic Roulette* (2007) or *Seeds of Deception* by Jeffrey M. Smith, or watch any of the many documentaries on the subject, including *GMO OMG*, *The World According to Monsanto*, and *Genetic Roulette*.

Nanotechnology

Nanotechnology refers to the manufacture of substances in extremely small measures. Technically speaking, a nanometre is one billionth of a metre. When nanotechnology meets food production, there's a potential problem. The substances that are injected into foods are so miniscule that they are being directly absorbed into the bloodstream.

Here's an example. One candy bar manufacturer has used nanotechnology in adding a preservative to the candy's coating to prevent spoiling. When you eat this candy bar, the preservative is absorbed directly into your bloodstream. We've talked about the dangers of preservatives and how they can be toxic. The issue here is that by going directly into the bloodstream, the toxins are bypassing even the smallest amount of filtering that would normally occur in the intestines and liver.

FOOD MILES

The distance it takes for the food we typically eat to travel from its place of origin to our supermarkets also presents problems. There's an impact on the environment, of course; freshness is another issue. The average dinner of an American, Canadian, and Australian travels between four and ten thousand miles to reach their table.

Consider, for example, that even though Australia grows oranges, they also consume orange juice from concentrate made with oranges grown in Florida, which were shipped somewhere with lower wages to process, possibly elsewhere to be packaged, then to Australia, where the juice is reconstituted and finally sold. That's a lot of miles and fossil fuels.

Now compare that to Australians going to a farmers' market, buying oranges, squeezing them into a juice, and indulging in that freshly squeezed orange juice. Quite a difference: a few steps versus thousands of miles, and fresh, natural juice loaded with vitamins and fibre versus concentrated, pasteurized, and reconstituted juice.

Now think about the package this orange juice is in and where the paper originated, the ink for the label, and even the equipment used to process and package the product. When you consider all these factors involved in a simple glass of orange juice, you'll begin to see how far much of our food travels, how long it takes to get to us because of processing, and how many resources are used—when you can simply take the orange in its natural, compostable skin, and juice it. Not only is the quality compromised in store-bought juice, but in providing it, large companies are being environmentally wasteful (transportation pollutions, packaging wastes, etc.) and taking away from the local community's revenue and sustainability.

Many fruits and vegetables are picked before they are ripe, packaged, shipped, gassed to ripen quickly, then transported to grocery stores. It's just not simple, and it is not a sustainable global practice.

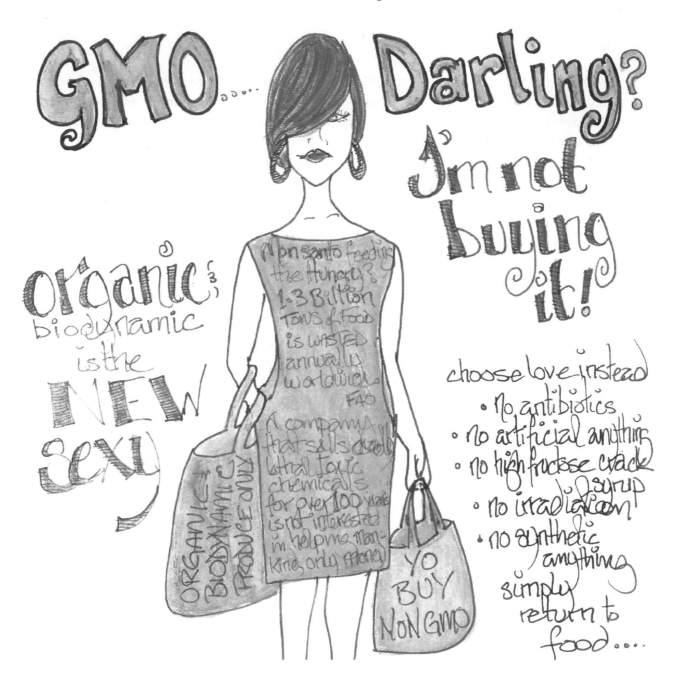

THEO FLEURY

When Theo Fleury came to work with me, he'd been suffering for years with pain and discomfort from Crohn's disease. After countless futile attempts to get better with the medical system, including having surgery to remove part of his gut, his intuition drew him to look at his diet.

When I first met him, I didn't know the significance of Theo's hockey career, nor of the years of suffering he'd experienced in many areas of his life. When he told me his age, I didn't believe him. I could have sworn he was ten years older. In fact, I asked him twice, because his age just didn't energetically compute.

After four months of working together, Theo and I did a segment on Calgary breakfast television to talk about how he no longer had pain since giving up the Lethal Recipe. We had been working online and by phone, so I hadn't seen him in person since we first met. When I saw him at the studio, I thought he was wearing makeup; his transformation was beyond his weight loss of forty pounds and putting Crohn's into remission. There was a vibrancy and colour in his face that was remarkable given the grey pallor of just months earlier. But he hadn't been to the makeup room. I was blown away by the contrast.

Theo had weaned himself off the Lethal Recipe and was living testimony to the power of returning to real food.

TWO COMMON MISCONCEPTIONS ABOUT HEALTHY EATING

When presented with the choice of eating well, many people believe one or both of these statements: "Eating healthy is time-consuming!" and "Eating well is too expensive."

These are misconceptions.

First, everyone on the planet has the same 24-hour clock. It's all about how you choose to spend your time. When you say you don't have enough time for something, you're essentially stating that it's not important enough to you to apportion any part of your 24 hours, 7 days a week, 52 weeks a year, 365 days a year to whatever it is. It is that simple. Whether it's a return to food, or your well-being in general, or you that *you* deem not valuable enough, the result is the same. You end up suffering.

When something is important, we find the time. If we have an incredibly busy day and someone we love is rushed to hospital with a life-threatening condition, we don't say, "I just need to finish this bit of work and keep this important meeting and will head straight over if I have any time left." We just don't do that. So instead we re-prioritize and move everything in our power to be there, and not because we can do anything about the situation, either—it is only a matter of what is most important.

But when it comes to our well-being, we take it for granted. Most of us are guilty of putting our health well down the list of priorities—until we are in a dire or life-threatening situation. Trust me, if you value your well-being and want to feel good, you have the time to make an effort to change things for the better.

Another common objection I get from people when it comes to eating well is that it is expensive. A client who flew me to the United States to do a lifestyle makeover was criticized by his colleagues for spending what it required to help me help him save his life. He was in a dire situation, but cognizant enough to know he needed help. At the end of our time, his justification for the expense was, "How much would I have paid for just one more day of life?"

Peter Menzel and Faith D'Aluisio's book, *Hungry Planet: What the World Eats* (2005), vividly illustrates that people in poorer countries—who live without expensive, packaged food—have fewer lifestyle diseases. Organic food and "food with integrity" cost more because they are worth more. But preparing meals from scratch still makes eating far more economical than eating conventional processed food. If processed food is cheaper than organic whole foods, the lower price is usually an indicator that there is no intrinsic goodness left in it. By and large, when it comes to our food, we get what we pay for. When it is important, we will find a way to get good food.

Debra Ross

Entrepreneur, socialite, and CEO of Gamma Tech Industries Debra Ross is an amazing whirlwind who does everything . Whereas most people in her position would have a cook and a maid, she fills those roles too—now, that is.

Before Debra flew me out to Calgary for a lifestyle makeover, I had her send me pictures of her fridge and cupboards. I asked her if she'd done a food audit without me, as her cupboards were barer than Old Mother Hubbard's. She said, "No, that's what they normally look like."

Here's what she has to say about our working together.

"Sherry came to my home for a complete overhaul of my eating and cooking habits. To my amazement, the change has been instant and obvious. Prior, I was beginning to suffer from all sorts of ailments and aches to the point of great concern. Please note that I did not cook … at all … until now. So this indeed is a HUGE change for me. Sherry's knowledge on the subject of health is extensive and yet she teaches at a level anyone could understand. Speaking to her client; not above them. I found her recipes easy to follow and all very tasty (a huge surprise to me). I feel amazing already and have no desire to ever go back to all the chemical overload my body had been existing in for so long. I can't wait to find out how I'll feel in a few months! So exciting.

"Sherry's passion is abundant and it's a pleasure to work with her. Best decision I have EVER made.

"Eternally grateful."
Debra Ross

DINOSAUR EGG PORRIDGE

We used to have toys in cereal; now the cereal is the toy—and just as nutritious. There are countless terrible, sugar-filled cereals on the grocery shelves. Let's choose one as an example. Quaker has a cereal called Dinosaur Eggs that claims to be a good source of calcium. The commercial shows that when you pour hot water onto the cereal, the dinosaur eggs hatch into baby dinosaurs. Now, what child wouldn't want that breakfast? The company then adds that its cereal is a good source of calcium. Convinced, the uninformed parent buys the cereal and feeds it to their beloved child daily, not realizing the truth about the product. They mistakenly think, "Hey, my kid loves it *and* it's good for them." But they're wrong and they don't even realize it.

The truth is, Dinosaur Eggs has 124 words on its ingredient list, most of them unpronounceable. This cereal is full of preservatives, dyes, artificial flavours, and other unhealthy ingredients. Yet the marketing is focused on making the consumer think it's a good source of calcium. The only thing this cereal is a good source of is chemicals.

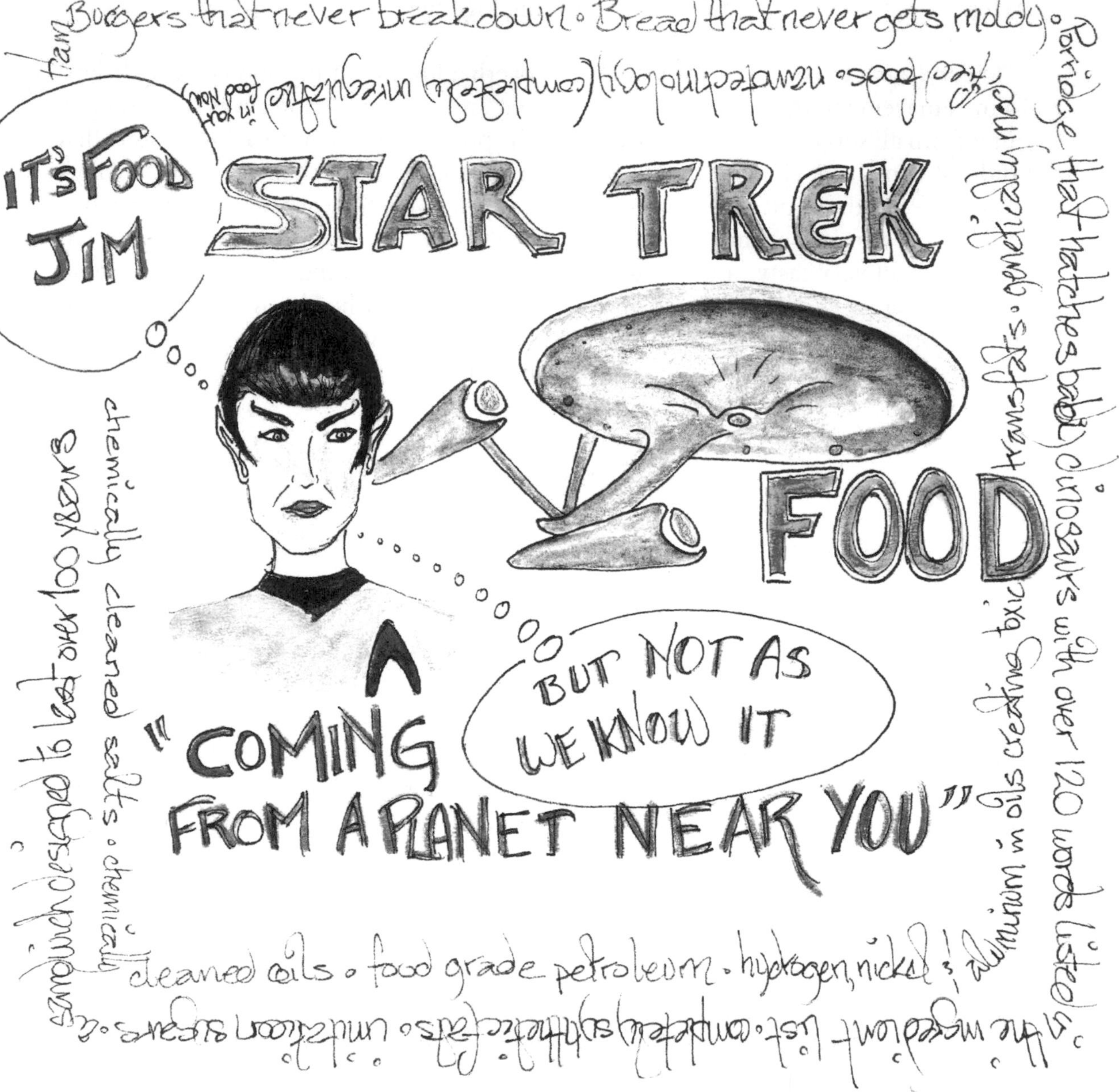
STAR TREK
FOOD
IT'S FOOD JIM
BUT NOT AS WE KNOW IT
"COMING FROM A PLANET NEAR YOU"
Burgers that never break down • Bread that never gets moldy •
Porridge that hatches baby dinosaurs with over 120 words listed in
the ingredient list • completely synthetic fats • imitation sugars •
sandwich designed to last over 100 years • chemically cleaned salts • chemically
cleaned oils • food grade petroleum • hydrogen, nickel &
aluminum in oils creating toxic transfats • genetically modified foods •
nanotechnology (completely unregulated in your food now) • ham

Please don't fall for this kind of ploy. Companies won't hesitate to say their product is a good part of a nutritious breakfast, but it's up to you to check out the ingredients. In 2012, Nutella was sued by a woman who saw that in spite of the product's claim to be nutritious, it contained 200 calories, 21 grams of sugar, and 11 grams of fat in two tablespoons alone. She won. Do your own research and use common sense, and you'll make smarter choices.

FOOD POLITICS

It is well documented that food manufacturers and the food industry have more power to have foods approved as safe for consumption than those who are qualified to evaluate their safety. Industry has more influence on what is approved for your health than anyone else. Otherwise, how on earth could they make cigarettes legal and raw milk illegal?

When you start to enter the maze of holistic nutritional information, it will astonish you. Many of the books in my resource section will illuminate you. If you have not seen information about how industry controls our food system, then you just haven't been looking.

You cannot trust the government or manufacturers to make decisions in your best interest. This is not a conspiracy theory—it just is what it is. But worrying or apportioning blame is a waste of energy—energy best diverted to taking protective, corrective action, and educating yourself so you know what is happening to your food. Then make decisions based on what you are prepared to invest in. What you choose to eat is in fact an investment in your present energy levels and the future of your health.

As you now see, millions of people think they are eating food when in fact they are not. Processed food is no longer real food. It can look, smell, and taste as though it is, but not only does it not truly nourish you, it is also toxic and addictive and is making people sick, fat, and exhausted. By now, you can say with me that the answer to this problem lies in returning to eating real food as close to its pristine, natural state as possible.

Never before have we had both the best of food and the worst of food simultaneously available to us. You can go into a supermarket and find food, food everywhere, and not a crumb to eat. And in the space of a mile, you can find a whole food market with more nourishing food than they will ever sell, much of it being wasted and thrown away.

The answer to this problem doesn't lie in tearing down food companies or blowing them up in a militant revolution. Many people believe that food companies are evil, and that we are powerless against them and what they decide to sell. The truth is, we've helped create the monsters, in buying from food companies that produce unnatural food, or nonfood. It can be frustrating to discover the big monster got so big—in part—because we unwittingly fed it. So stop feeding the monster and it will starve. Ask companies to make good-quality natural food, without chemicals (and to be willing to invest in it), and don't buy their products otherwise. You could also start shopping at the farmers' markets or at stores that stock food from local farmers who ethically produce organic foods.

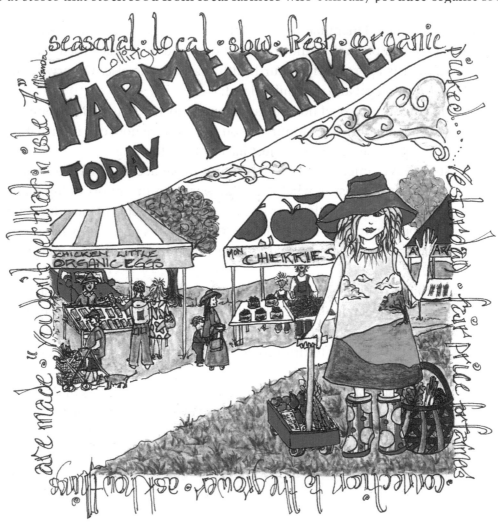

CHAPTER THREE

NATURE'S PRINCIPLE

"Nature does nothing uselessly."
Aristotle

NATURE'S PRINCIPLE OF HOW WE ARE MEANT TO EAT

Even the most earnest students and teachers of nutrition are confused by the rules, so how does that bode for those who don't have the luxury of taking years out of their life to study nutrition? That was my thinking when I used to subscribe to journals of clinical nutrition and I read peer-reviewed-and-validated studies that contradicted findings of other "credible" studies. I saw report after report touting the benefits of products that contain ingredients that are known carcinogens.

How could anyone know what they are meant to be eating? I've been working in the nutrition field for almost thirty years, and just the other day I bought a new brand of sour dried cherries only to open them, taste them, and spit them out. When I read the ingredient list and saw refined sugar, I was annoyed with myself for not having checked before I bought them; I should know better after all this time. Then again, how sad that I have to look at the ingredient list of something that should have only one ingredient in it—sour cherries.

The constant contradiction, the unnatural ingredients, and the extreme processing of our food are essentially what drove me to the idea of returning to nature and traditional ways of gathering and thinking about food.

Nature's Principle is that **nature tells us what we are meant to eat, when to eat it, and the quantities we are meant to eat—all we have to do is observe how prolific the food is in nature, when it is obtainable in nature, and how difficult it is to obtain.**

Think about the nutrient on which we are most dependent, without which we cannot survive

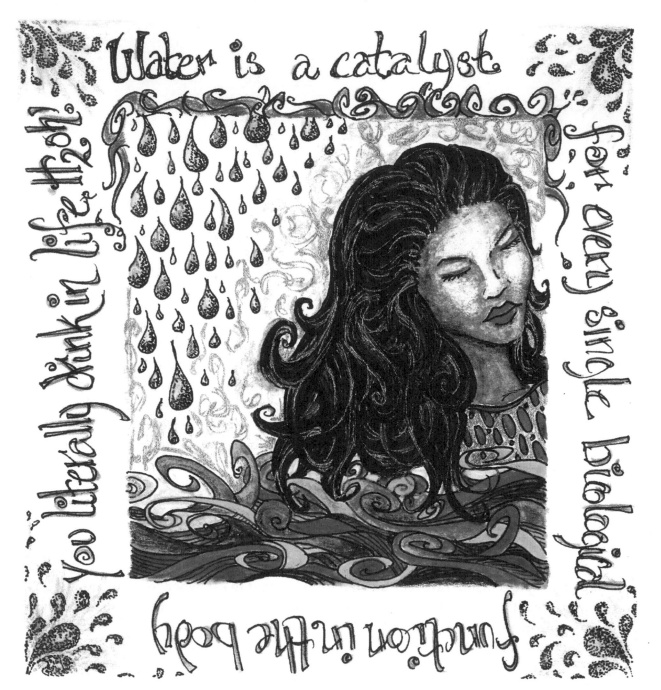

Water is a catalyst for every single biological function in the body. You literally drink in life H2oh!

long. It is the most abundant nutrient on the planet for humans, and most people take it so much for granted that they don't even think of it as a nutrient. In fact, most of my nutrition students do not answer correctly when I ask them what it could be, as they've not been taught that it is a nutrient. The answer is air. The definition of a nutrient is "a substance that provides nourishment essential for growth and the maintenance of life."

We depend most on air. It is, arguably, the most important nutrient essential to our growth—we cannot survive many minutes without it. Conveniently, it is also the most abundant nutrient on earth. Isn't it nice that you don't have to wake up each morning and wonder where to get your air from?

The next most essential nutrient for growth and maintenance of life for humans—something we cannot go many days without—is water. It covers 70 percent of the planet, and is the second most abundant nutrient on the *planet*.

There is a compositional equivalent of this nutrient in our bodies. Typically, they are 70 percent water. Most thriving cultures settle in areas close to potable water. We are now learning what our intuition has told us all along—that the best water comes from springs, and when we chemically clean and treat our water, in the ways most tap water is treated, it not only tastes bad, but it is also not as hydrating. Spring water is smooth, sweet, and compelling to drink, whereas tap water feels often like hard work. This is why there has been such a revival of people drinking spring water; they even hunt for it and carry large quantities of it down mountains in glass bottles from springs where the water is pushed up by aquifers.

The third most abundant source of nutrients that humans depend on covers a great deal of the earth and is green, or at least stems from green vegetation. The majority of the nutrients come from plants that have pulled macronutrients and micronutrients from their seeds, the sun, and the soil. There are more varieties of vegetation than any other food we eat. It is at ground level. We don't have to trap it or catch it, and most of it can be eaten with little preparation or cooking.

For years we have been told that we are meant to eat more vegetables than fruit, mostly with the nutritional reasoning that vegetables are more nutrient-dense and lower in calories. But nature tells us this in a different way that makes more sense, in that there are many more species of vegetables than of fruit.

Vegetables are the easiest foods to obtain and can be eaten raw or cooked. By and large, they are most healthy when they are young, fresh, raw, organic, whole, and as found in nature, closest to where they have been picked.

Next, we look at fruit. As I said earlier, there are fewer fruit species than vegetable species. If you plant a vegetable seed and a fruit seed, the vegetable seed will produce food faster.[9] Plant a broccoli seed and you have sprouts in days; wait a few months and you have food. If you plant an apple seed, it takes years to grow a tree that produces fruit. Typically, you wait until it ripens, and then you are rewarded with sweetness, beautiful colours, fresh fragrance and full flavour, all of which develops during the ripening process, when most of the nutrients are infused into the plant. The added bonus is that once you finally get to that stage, it is pretty much "fast food."

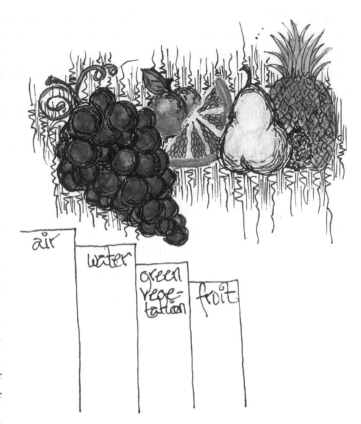

That said, fruitarians living in the Midwest of North America are not living according to the hierarchy of nature that informs us how best to eat. Often, the blood work of fruitarians reveals enormous amounts of fructose. Even natural sugars can overload the pancreas. There are also many fruitarians who lose their teeth over an extended time, due to excess sugar.

Where in the world have traditional cultures eaten only fruit year round? Where in nature does fruit grow 365 days a year? Is that the only type of vegetation that grows there? Even if there are such areas, they cannot sustain everyone living there drawing their only food from that region. Fruit trees take a great deal more resources from the earth in comparison to vegetables.

This summary gives you part of the typical hierarchy of nature's provisions. The availability of some foods and water may depend on your geographical location or on your country's economic status or other factors. However, especially in developed countries, where we are faced with countless processed foods, we can hopefully see Nature's Principle readily at work and be able to make our return to food.

Next, we could look at grains, pulses, nuts, seeds, and spices, which we do in depth in the *Return to Food* Program. But for now, consider what things and how things grow in nature. Compare that to what you eat and to how much of what you eat is abundant in nature or unobtainable in nature. The farther away from nature your food originates, the less vitality it will have. Definitely food for thought.

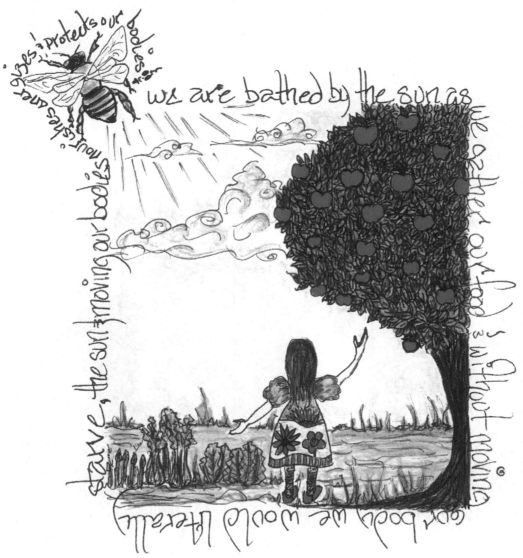

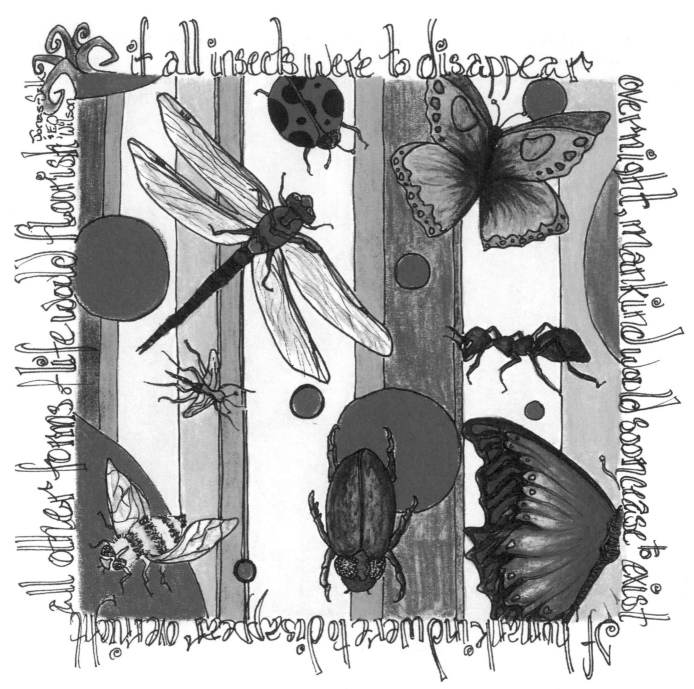

If all insects were to disappear overnight, Mankind would soon cease to exist. If mankind were to disappear, overnight all other forms of life would flourish.

Jonas Salk / EO Wilson

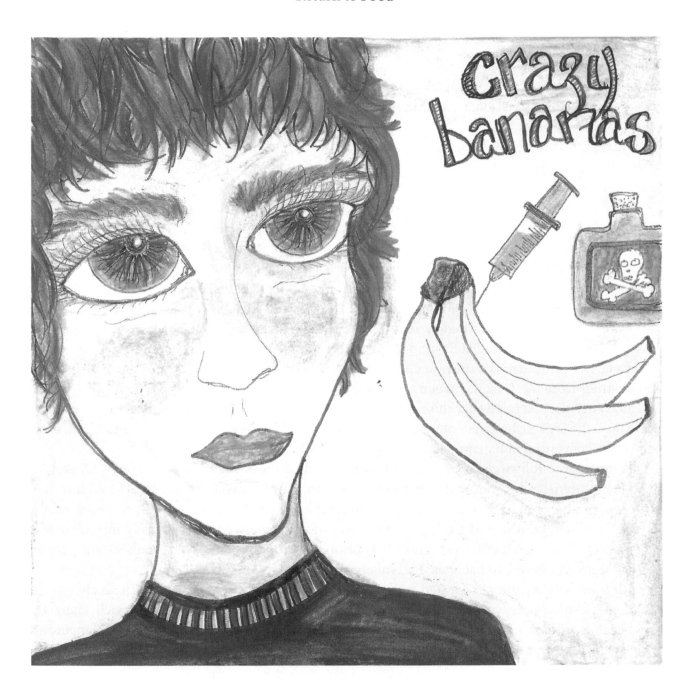

PESTICIDES: THE BANANA STORY

Let me tell you about my experience with pesticides. In 1993, I started a cooking school in Australia. I wanted a different twist on a cooking school, so I chose to make it an organic-focused cooking school.

Up to that time in my life I was convinced that I was allergic to bananas. Every time I ate just a bit of one, I became ill with stomach cramps, nausea, and heartburn. Of course, it wasn't pleasant, and I vowed to avoid bananas for life.

During one of my cooking classes, I had a recipe that called for bananas, so I had bunches of organic ones. For some odd reason, I felt compelled to eat a banana. I knew it would make me sick and I'd regret it, but I just couldn't resist it that day, so I ate it. It tasted so incredibly delicious, I ate a second. I didn't care at that point if I was facing excruciating pain.

But what happened—or didn't happen—amazed me. I didn't get ill. Not at all. I was convinced I was over my "banana allergy." Not long afterwards, I was at a social function and I had a banana. Soon after eating it, I was stunned by stomach cramps and nausea, the same painful stomach problems I'd had before. I immediately made the connection: the banana wasn't organic.

Years later, I came across a study of chimps at the Copenhagen Zoo. The chimps normally peeled and ate their bananas. One day when they were given organic bananas, they ate them whole, skin and all. When they were given a choice between organic bananas and non-organic ones. Each time, they chose the organic bananas, ate them whole and only when the organic ones were finished, they peeled the conventional bananas and left the peel.

This story came full circle for me last year when I visited the Northey Street Farmers' Market in Brisbane, Queensland. I met with a banana seller who grew biodynamic bananas. I told him my problem with the fruit and asked if he knew anyone else who had a similar experience. He assured me it was quite common and explained that conventional banana growers actually inject banana stalks with poison used to kill white ants. This poison goes into the bananas and makes some people quite ill. I wasn't allergic to bananas; I was allergic to the poisonous chemicals.

If our food isn't organic, it's treated with pesticides, fungicides, and herbicides. These chemicals leach into the food or leave residue on it after harvest. Strawberries, bell peppers, spinach, cherries, and peaches are among the foods that contain the highest levels of chemicals. These dangerous toxins have been linked to cancer, Alzheimer's, neurological impairments, and even birth defects.

Biodynamic produce contains higher levels of nutrients than organic produce. Biodynamic farmers employ elaborate, natural methods that work to build up the integrity and health of the soil. They are a wonderful example of working with nature to maximize its potential and power. This is in direct contrast to thinking that we can outsmart nature and improve upon it. No one becomes a biodynamic farmer to get rich quick. They choose that form of farming out of integrity and with ideologies that are completely at odds with corporate farming.

THE SOIL STORY: GETTING TO THE ROOT OF THE PROBLEM

Anyone who says there's no nutritional benefit in organic farming over conventional farming does not know how plants obtain nutrients. In a handful of healthy soil, there are over eight billion micro-organisms that work synergistically to provide nutrients to the plants. Those eight billion micro-organisms have their own little universe and, if that universe is healthy, the plants that are grown in it will get what they need to naturally ward off diseases and predators. No chemicals needed.

The healthier the ecology of the soil, the more nutrients it can provide, which in turn creates a stronger, more robust plant with higher amounts of vitamins, minerals, and phytonutrients that it can pass on to us. Sadly, what often happens is that crops are grown in the same soil year after year, and nutrients are not replenished. Thus, the soil is depleted. In addition, when chemicals are added to a plant to ward off predators and disease, a host of problems results. The toxins on the surface of the plant don't stay there. Rain washes them into the soil, where they begin to kill micro-organisms. Many of these pesticides are designed to disable the nervous system of insects, which is not too dissimilar to the human nervous system. Imagine what it would do to fragile micro-organisms. Our plants grow in this and they, like the soil, lack nutrients.

The manufactured chemicals sprayed on crops and into the soils are highly toxic. Billions of pounds of these chemicals are sold around the world and used on our food annually. The US Environmental Protection Agency (EPA) reports about 300,000 illnesses each year from pesticide use. Over 100,000 people die of cancer related to pesticides annually, over 17,000 of them in China. In the developing world, it's estimated that 3 million workers each year experience severe poisoning and, of those, 18,000 die. More than 5 billion pounds of soil chemicals are used globally, much of which ends up in our food and waterways.[10] Chemicals impact our health every day, most of the time without us even knowing. Women in the eighth week of their pregnancy who live near farms sprayed with pesticides are several times more likely to miscarry. Researchers have found over three hundred chemicals in the umbilical cord blood of newborns.[11]

Eighty thousand different farming chemicals are used in the United States. Two hundred of these have been tested as safe; five are regulated by the EPA. In 2012, the chemical industry spent $56 million dollars on lobbying for the use of their products.

None of these chemicals belong in our food, homes, bodies, or planet. It is time to stop feeding this monster and to start loving the earth.

Anyone who says there's no nutritional difference between organic and conventional produce simply does not understand how a plant grows and is nourished.

A Quick Reference Guide to Types of Growing

- Conventional—grown with chemicals and synthetic and organic fertilizers.
- Organic—grown primarily without chemicals; non-GMO.
- Biodynamic—a growing system developed by Dr. Rudolf Steiner that works at building up the integrity and health of the soil through many elaborate and labour-intensive practices.
- Hydroponic—plants grown without the use of soil. It is possible to grow hydroponically without the use of chemicals, but it is much harder and rarely implemented commercially.

Corporate Organic versus True Organic

Once again, I come back to the concept of eating according to nature, trusting your intuition, and listening to your body when it comes to selecting foods that will nourish your body and soul, for you and your family.

This applies to considering "organic" foods, too. As I've mentioned earlier, big business, which sells almost all the foods in grocery stores, is out to make a profit. This is their number one goal. They will take advantage of the consumer, manipulate words and data, and use clever, often misleading marketing to sell their product. They do this at any cost.

When you go to the grocery store and see a section filled with foods labelled "organic," you naturally assume these foods are healthy and good for you. Unfortunately, this isn't necessarily true. We must think about eating according to nature when shopping for organics, too. Again, the least processed food—meaning, the closest the food is to how it's found in nature—is the best food for you. This holds true for organic as well as conventionally grown food.

Unfortunately, a food labelled organic can still be highly refined and exposed to or actually contain chemicals. Maybe the potatoes in a bag of organic potato chips were farmed organically, but then the manufacturer used unhealthy oils, chemicals, and preservatives to take that potato through extreme processing to make it into a chip. That organic chip is not healthy in this case.

Organic yogurt is another example. One may think, "Oh, this is organic yogurt. It must be good for me." However, many low-fat organic yogurts contain upwards of 40 percent sugar and are no healthier than ice cream.

You're more likely to find true organic, healthy foods from local producers to whom you can put a name and face, and where you can find accountability. The CEO of a food manufacturer located thousands of miles away from you is less likely to feel connected to consumers and, therefore, would probably find it easier to make decisions without fully appreciating the impact of his or her choices. I've developed distrust in multinational food companies—in fact, any food company whose intention to make money is their primary motivator. Producing food of integrity requires time, patience, care, and passion, things that in the corporate world add cost to the bottom line, because they cannot easily be manufactured and streamlined.

A local farmer knows that his customers live in his town; maybe his kids go to school with yours, you attend the same church, his granddad grew up with your grandma, and so on. This farmer wants to make you happy, keep you satisfied, and ideally cares about his customers' well-being. To this end, he needs to operate with integrity. Kinesthetically, you will feel it. When a farmer grows with integrity, it's palpable when you hold, feel, and eat this kind of food.

When you source your food locally, you minimize your carbon footprint dramatically and contribute to the well-being of your own community. Our food system is incredibly complex; eating local comes with its own complications—for instance, what if the local food is not organic but you could buy organic from California? There is no quick-fix solution to that, but eating locally can start with herbs in a pot growing on your windowsill.

If for some reason you don't have the ability to source locally for produce, dairy, meats, or other food, you can still research companies that produce and sell true organic dairy, meat, and produce.

Find out their company mission and gauge their integrity. With the internet and easy, immediate access to heaps of information, this should only take a few minutes to do. Then make your buying decisions based on companies that you feel are supporting the values you believe in too.

Humans have been highly adaptable to their environments—the sustainability of biodiversity depends on it. If you look at the traditional diet of the Inuit in the Arctic (compared to people on the Standard American Diet) who survive with few lifestyle diseases in the absence of fruit year round, little vegetation, and with up to 50 percent fat as the mainstay of their diet, you can see a story emerging that defies what many modern nutrition experts are saying—that is, that there is a universal diet for the planet. This is simply not true. Our bodies are adapted according to our environment, and the planet's prosperity and biodiversity depends on species eating in accordance to the nature of their environment, not half the globe away.

Nature is constantly communicating with us, but for the better part of the last one hundred to two hundred years we've disconnected from the innate intelligence in our food, so we miss out on what it tells us. Sadly, not fully understanding the complexities of our natural environment, we think we can improve on nature, to conform it to what suits us. Instead, without fully understanding the ramifications of changing even one thing, we've created many problems for all species.

"Look deep into nature, and then you will understand everything better."
Albert Einstein

The Power of Plant Foods

When plants (fruits and vegetables; nuts, seeds, and beans) are grown organically or biodynamically, without the use of chemicals, they are ideal for us. Packed with vitamins, minerals, fats, fibres, phytochemicals, glyconutrients, and even electromagnetic energy, these foods offer our bodies a powerhouse of health benefits.

Vitamins help us produce energy, regulate tissue growth, protect cells from damage, keep our bones and teeth strong, heal properly, boost our immune system, and so much more. The body cannot make vitamins on its own; we must provide ourselves with them through our food. All the vitamins humans require for life (with the exception of B12) are found abundantly in the variety of plant foods nature offers.

Minerals

Unlike vitamins, which are organic and produced by vegetables, minerals come from the soil and are then absorbed by the plants we eat. We need minerals for many body processes, and most minerals possess multiple benefits. For example, calcium works to keep our bones strong and supports nerve transmission, iron helps the formation of hemoglobin and acts as an oxygen carrier, and magnesium relaxes the nervous system and helps alkalinize the body.

Together, vitamins and minerals work in many ways and are then absorbed by the plant to keep our bones and teeth strong, to support cell growth and development, and to help our organs and cells function optimally. Some minerals actually require certain vitamins to be able to work well. For example, calcium is often paired with vitamin D because the vitamin helps us absorb the mineral.

Fats

It's a myth that all fats are bad for us. This is one of the most commonly misunderstood nutrition facts. Fats found in their natural state are some of the healthiest nutrients around. Among other reasons, we need fats for energy, for the proper functioning of our brain and nerves, and to help transport fat-soluble vitamins, like vitamin D, through the body.

Fats from plant foods such as avocados, nuts, seeds, olives, and beans can substantially improve your health. A vital part of our daily nutrition, these fats can actually help us burn fat, to a point. Of course, excess nutrients consumed in unnatural amounts, even if they are natural, are not good for us. The fats to avoid particularly, however, are trans fats and saturated fats—those that have been produced by the Lethal Recipe.

The fats more easily obtained in nature are best for us. Think of consuming nuts and seeds before the oils made from them. Think of a whole avocado, and even better, coconut oil, as it requires less processing than avocado oil; coconut oil over butter; butter over margarine. Ask yourself, "Which is most easily sourced?" and if you are an environmentalist, "Which is produced with the least amount of water and the fewest food miles?" The answers are going to vary depending on where you live in the world and, admittedly, raises more questions than this book has space for.

Check out www.returntofood.com/fats for videos I've created on this topic.

Fibre

Consuming the proper amount of fibre in your daily diet is vital to your body's process of eliminating wastes and toxins. This function is, of course, essential to good health.

Plant foods offer a rich source of fibre the body can immediately use to stay regular and rid itself of toxic matter. Along with the fibre comes a wealth of other health benefits, such as lowering cholesterol and helping to regulate blood sugar levels.

Phytonutrients

Phytonutrients, originally called phytochemicals, are specific nutrients with disease-preventing properties, and protect our cells found naturally in plants. They derive from the flavour, colour, and aroma compounds, and are categorized in groups that include antioxidants, carotenoids, flavonoids, polyphenols, and more. This provides us with good reason to consume a wide range of colours in plant matter. Some of the more familiar phytochemicals are lycopene, caffeine, theobromine, betacarotene, lutein, capsaicin, tannic acid, resveratrol, and rutin.

To date, scientists have catalogued tens of thousands of phytochemicals that are essential for protection from sickness and disease. Plant foods grown organically or biodynamically have been proven to be significantly higher in phytonutrients—which makes sense when we understand how a plant grows and obtains these compounds.

Wild Foods and Genetic Superiority

As you now know, the less altered a food is, the closer it remains to its wild state and the higher in vital nutrients it is.

There is a great deal of marketing hype around the relatively new term "superfoods," referring to substances such as goji berries, açai berries, mangosteen, and even chocolate. The media have created a kind of craze for superfoods. Now, for convenience especially, people are eating huge, unnatural amounts of them in powdered forms. They are filling themselves with dehydrated versions of a range of superfoods and sometimes excluding other crucial foods from their diets. They mistakenly think, and are often led to believe, that consuming these superfoods—despite what

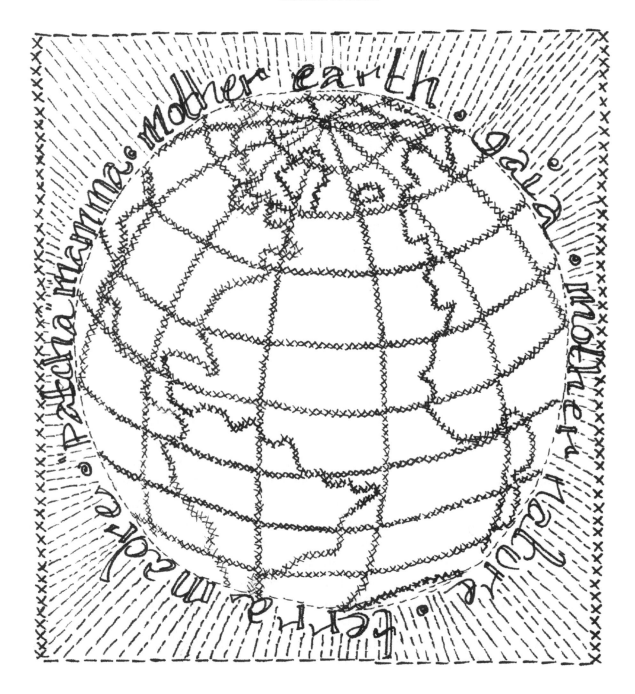

other highly processed foods they put into their bodies—will make them healthy, save them from sickness and disease, and even help them lose weight. I believe there is a need for caution and wisdom here.

Henry David Thoreau said, *"A weed is simply a plant whose virtues have not yet been discovered."*

I say, *"A superfood is simply a plant whose virtues have been discovered."*

Dehydrated foods are great for times when you can't get the fresh version, but they lack valuable water content and living energy. As we talk about sourcing our foods as nature intended, considering the Consumption Concept, the amount of superfoods consumed in dehydrated or powdered form can be far greater than we would ever consume if we were gathering foods ourselves in nature. We can eat in a matter of weeks what would take months to source in nature. Eating out of balance with nature can create imbalance in our bodies.

Living Naturally in an Unnatural World

The challenge with Nature's Principle is fitting it into the context of the modern world. We don't eat naturally anymore because our lives and food systems are so far away from what is natural. So how do we transition to living naturally in our unnatural world?

We need to address the biggest obstacle to our achieving this. The problem is the modern supermarket. It presents us with this dilemma: what is most abundant, most easily consumed, and most compelling and addictive to consume is also the easiest and cheapest to obtain, if you count your food preparation time. These are foods that require enormous amounts of energy, both of human and land resources, and the foods we should be eating in small amounts. But it's all too accessible and convenient. How can Nature's Principle compete?

Knowledge. When you know how real food affects and empowers you and what are its long-term benefits, and you desire a better quality of life, you can make the right decisions toward change, both for yourself and the planet.

In nature, convenience is a natural protective mechanism in that the most easily obtained and readily available foods are the most nutritious. On the give-take scale, they give more nutrients than anti-nutrients, which are natural or synthetic compounds that prevent the absorption of nutrients. Today, the foods most readily available are completely the opposite. While many are making the move to growing their own food or developing community plots, most people in developed countries still do not have gardens or plots of land on which to grow their own food; and in supermarkets, the most convenient foods are the ones that are not only highest in energy (calories) but also lowest in nutrients and cost. Think candies, one-dollar burgers, and soft drinks. We also have "family-sized" or "club-sized" packaging to make it cheaper to buy large amounts of mostly processed food.

Our natural inclination to make our lives easier was once rewarded with the protection and nourishment of real food. That natural inclination has translated over the centuries into laziness that is now contributing to alarming death rates associated with lifestyle diseases. Once upon a time, having a garden was a huge time-saving factor, because you didn't have to go out and forage for your food. Today, people complain about even having to chop vegetables for a meal.

Less than sixty years ago, the average amount of time spent preparing the evening meal was six hours. Today, it is thirty minutes, and even then, I get many clients who say it is all too hard. While I believe they are genuinely stressed, the problem is in the way we choose to spend our time and what we prioritize. The easier life chores become for us, the higher the expectations we have for life to become even easier. For those of you who are old enough, remember the excitement of getting your first dishwasher? Back then, it was going to save so much time, and perhaps now you think what an annoyance it is to have to load and empty it.

It is reminiscent of how Jane Jetson in the 1970s futuristic cartoon *The Jetsons* complained about how irritating it was (rolling her eyes and sighing) that she actually had to press a button to do her ironing. I wonder just how far our efforts to make life easier will go and what we will get used to, and to what detriment. I say all this with the full admission of being prone to laziness and often avoiding housework, even with all the modern conveniences available. The point is simply to put things into perspective.

The more you think about Nature's Principle, the more figuring out what is good for us and making good choices just falls into place, and the harder it is to be swayed by the multimillion-dollar manipulation by companies through media. Using Nature's Principle is a way of cutting through nutritional confusion and inconsistencies. This is not about science now. It is to provoke thought, and to question how far we have deviated from eating naturally over the past one hundred years.

Returning to nature and eating naturally can now seem counterintuitive, awkward, and unnatural, even though nothing could be better for us. The same adaptive evolutionary process that worked in our favour in nature works against us when it comes to industrialized food choices. In nature, human neophobia toward food made us cautious about eating something that could potentially make us sick or kill us. Over thousands of years, cultures developed the ability to identify substances that were edible and also medicinal as well as lethal or harmful. That information was passed down so we had knowledge combined with experience to source food that was good, healthy, and life-giving.

But in the way that a domesticated or human-fed wild animal no longer knows how to survive in the wild, we too have lost our connection to nature. We've relinquished trust in ourselves and given it over to those who provide our food. The supermarket was designed to feed millions without the threat of food poisoning due to the myriad complications that can come about from mass agriculture, farming, processing, and manufacturing. Now we have a hyper-hygienic, sanitized food system. We do our best to remove any living elements from our food to prevent instantaneous food poisoning, while allowing chemicals and extreme processing. However, this changes the molecular structure of our foods so that they are indeed poisonous—except that they poison us slowly, so that we don't notice we're being poisoned. The many chemicals are in such low doses that we are rarely struck down immediately, which makes it difficult to differentiate what is causing the itching, twitching, drowsiness, irritability, headache, runny nose, shortness of breath, heartburn, nausea, sneezing, and numerous other ways your body is trying to communicate to you that something is amiss. Going to a chemist to buy a highly processed drug to treat our symptoms, which often creates its own set of problems called "side effects," is now considered normal, but it's hardly natural.

CHAPTER FOUR

THE CONSUMPTION CONCEPT

*You would eat completely differently if you had to source
your own food in nature.*

THE CONSUMPTION CONCEPT

If we had to source our food in nature, even the most healthy and environmentally sensitive of us would be eating very differently than we are now. I know it is true for me and most of my colleagues, friends, and students. Chances are this is true for you, unless you are already growing and sourcing all of your food.

The Consumption Concept bleeds into every area of life and is a way of rethinking our relationship with food.

Eating outside of what you can and would source for yourself is not a new issue for man. That everyone ate well and naturally in the olden days is a fallacy. The Egyptians, for example, sourced food for their nobility and royalty. Often slaves, they grew, harvested, husked, and ground the grain, sourced honey, and found anything else the elite wanted. Thus, the privileged ate however much they desired. It would have taken them a great deal of time to source their food themselves, and in doing so, they would have worked off much more of its energy. But even when people are active, too much food, albeit natural, can cause harm. This is why autopsies of pharaohs and Egyptian nobility show incidences of tooth decay, diabetes, and other lifestyle-related ailments. By contrast, the peasants who had access to simple food and a clean environment rarely had these diseases of excess; they were more likely to suffer from malnourishment than from lifestyle diseases. Even natural foods consumed outside a natural context can create imbalance.

Many think of farms as natural ways of getting food, but this is not necessarily true. Cropping and monoculture are man-made constructs. Most stretches of land that are farmed today with one crop were once home to thousands of species of plants, insects, and animals living in an ecosystem and cycle wherein one species became the food for another. In this ecosystem, every species' waste was food or building materials for another. We are the only species on the planet that creates garbage. We no longer offer up our bodies for food for other species when we die. We are buried in a box to keep things out or we are cremated, which—given the toxic nature of the food most people are eating today that then comprises the contents of their cells—is probably the wiser choice, environmentally speaking.

It may come as a big surprise, but even many raw food converts are eating unnaturally, consuming foods in amounts they could never possibly source in their natural environment. Though their food is real and natural—providing it's organic—the copious amounts they eat (for whatever reason, such as not balancing variety and the body thus wanting more, or thinking that more is better) create imbalance in the body. I've seen people eat large amounts of raw cashews, seeds, and other nuts beyond what they could possibly source naturally. Health issues and symptoms of imbalance result, such as halitosis and insulin resistance to pancreatic cancer from too much sugar in fruit.

As we learned earlier, this also happens when people go crazy for superfoods or medicinals. Medicinal plants were once used to prevent and heal disease or other ailments. Yet I've seen superfood enthusiasts eating medicinals as though they are food, often with dozens of other concentrated, nutrient-dense foods. Traditionally, tribal medicine men and women used medicinals strategically and intuitively, knowing the person and local environment, and taking that into consideration when prescribing treatment. Even in their natural, unadulterated form, medicinals require us to be intelligent and intuitive, to listen to our body when we take them. They are not necessarily meant to be consumed every day of the year, or long-term, without thought and checking in to see contraindications and how they impact the body.

Chocolate Cake from Scratch

Eating a piece of simple chocolate cake takes about ten minutes, if you are taking your time and savouring every bite. It takes about a half-hour to make the cake from a box and an hour to do it "from scratch." Making a cake from scratch nowadays is enough to deter even keen cake eaters.

Now imagine making a chocolate cake when you have to source your own ingredients. You have to grow and harvest the wheat, hull the grains from the husk and then dry and grind them, and then sieve out the most nutritious parts to make white flour. Then you need some cacao. You travel to South America, get the pods from the cacao tree, extract the nibs from the pods, grind the nibs, and separate the cacao from the butter and liquor.

Perhaps you can find some vanilla beans on the way back, in Mexico, which is the second most expensive spice in the world after saffron, because growing it is labour-intensive. From pollinating to making true vanilla, it takes over a year. Processing the beans involves curing, kilning, drying in the sun for months, conditioning, and grading them. Making the result into vanilla extract involves several other processes. These you can still do in a relatively natural environment, unlike with artificial vanilla, which is synthetically produced from a polymer that is a by-product of wood pulp being broken down using sulfites or sulfates; it could not be made in nature.

On your way back home from Mexico, you're going to want to find some cane juice, or you can create your sugar from beets (keeping in mind it is more labour-intensive to make sugar from beets). There are about fourteen steps in making beet sugar to get it to the refined or even brown stage that most people use to make cakes. We haven't even got to sourcing the milk or butter yet, but at least they're the easier ingredients to procure.

So, you get the picture, right? What would your chocolate cake look like if you had to source and create it from scratch in nature? How long would it take and how much appreciation would you have for the precious finished product? Would you have a different relationship with chocolate cake than if you bought it in your local bakery? Keep in mind that what I've listed is a far more innocent ingredient compilation than the average cake from your average bakery.

You can see that nature has inbuilt protective mechanisms against obesity. You would work off way more calories creating the cake from "nature's scratch" than you would ever get from eating it. Understanding the resources required by the earth and humans to create a food gives you an insight into how much you're meant to be eating of it.

Really thinking about the Miss Piggy quote "Never eat more than you can lift," I realize that, in a sense, she had a grasp of the Consumption Concept long before I did.

PICK YOUR POISONS

Don't get me wrong. As much as I believe chocolate cake is not a health food, I also believe, as Benjamin Franklin did about beer, that chocolate is God's way of saying he loves us and wants us to be happy. The same goes for wine, a great cup of coffee, and bacon. I'm not saying you can never, ever eat any of these processed foods. You can pick your poisons, but don't forget about the accumulative effect. The body can cope with a certain amount of toxins—it has mechanisms in place for such things—provided that the bulk of what we are doing is highly nourishing, energizing, and protective. But the more toxins we ingest, put on our skin in the form of beauty and cleaning products, inhale, take as pills, and absorb as toxins from the environment, the more these toxins collectively accumulate in our systems and the greater the potential they have to make us sick.

Remember two things about this.

One—many of the so-called health foods are toxic to the body; the way they are made is so far away from nature that in fact they will make the body sick.

Two—the thoughts we think, just like the food we eat, can be toxic or they can have the power to nourish, energize, and protect the body. So, too, when given only a choice of bad food to eat, try to think the most positive thoughts you can while eating it. There is a growing body of evidence to prove that how we eat, the social context in which we eat, is as powerful as what we eat. Remember what I said in Chapter One: eat with love and enjoyment, not guilt or stress. Emotions affect our digestive systems and hormone production, so let go and enjoy the food.

I would much rather eat a greasy bowl of noodles with people who are loving, positive, and nonjudgmental, than have the most nutritious, gourmet, home-prepared meal with people who are angry, depressed, and negative. There is limited value in becoming obsessive about the quality of the food you eat and about your health while neglecting a cancerous personality.

You need to clean your body before you can truly trust its signals. In the meantime, listen to how you feel after you have eaten a food and to how you feel when you remove something from your diet.

The Chicken or the Egg

If I were to ask you what you would like for dinner tonight, a meal made from chicken or a meal made from eggs, what would you choose? When I do this in my seminars, an overwhelming 85 to 90 percent say they'll have chicken. Statistics back this up: chicken consumption in 2014 for North Americans is around eighty-three pounds.[12]

Now what if you were given the same choice in nature—that is to say, as with the chocolate cake above, you have to source your own ingredients? If you were having an omelette, what would you do? You'd go out into nature, maybe your own backyard, and gather some eggs.

If you were sourcing for the chicken dinner, you'd have to catch a chicken (not an easy task!), kill, pluck, bleed, disembowel, disassemble, and prepare it.

Considering both of these options, if I were to ask you again what dinner you would choose, I'm guessing that you, just like the audiences in my seminars, would then choose an egg dish. In fact, when I ask how many would become vegetarian if they had to kill their own meat, many hands go up, including mine.

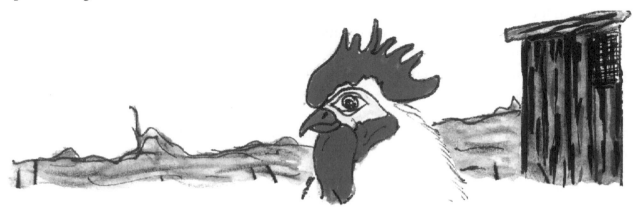

Consider, too, that in a natural environment, killing a chicken, at least a laying hen, would mean that a source of eggs for months or even years would now be gone, in one meal.

When I told this story in one of my Holistic Food Preparation classes, Chlotilda, a bright student from Kenya, said, "We are chicken farmers and even we kill a chicken for a meal for ourselves only once a month or every six weeks, and even then we invite other families to share the meal."

Chicken is consumed on such a regular basis in the Western world that it's hard to imagine that not too long ago, it was a special dinner reserved for only once a year, at Christmas. Today, chicken is consumed on a regular basis in the Western world; it's a commonplace meal. In fact, I've had clients tell me they have chicken more than ten times a week. They eat something for breakfast with chicken in it, a chicken sandwich for lunch, and then they have it again for dinner. This happens day after day. And keep in mind that this is typically low-quality, undernourished chicken, nowhere near the organic, free-range chicken.

Chicken meat is an intensively farmed product today. In conventional farming, the chickens often live in unnatural, filthy conditions indoors, causing disease and, in hot weather, mass death. Chemicals are used in their processing, in their feed, and injected into their bodies. They are sometimes forcefed in order to get them to grow faster. Today's chicken is a far cry from how chicken a hundred years ago was raised and processed. (Not to mention the environmental impact of how chicken is produced today.)

Chickens are naturally hens of the forest, and before breeding for mass consumption, their meat was dark and in comparison tough. For a master class I did called "Chicken, the new white meat," I researched for weeks the now standard practices in the conventional chicken-processing industry and how they have created a massive environmental hazard. What and how they feed the birds is completely unnatural and is often passed to us, the consumers. The scope of this industry is too much for this book, but you can research it yourself—if you dare. It's not for the faint of heart.

All of this leads us back—yet again!—to the same simple concept: if you want optimal health, keep your eating as close to nature as possible. Consider what you'd eat if you had to source it yourself. With this vital principle in mind—and adhered to—you won't need charts, scientific data, food pyramids, or even the advice of a nutritionist or doctor to eat healthfully and live disease-free.

The Consumption Concept and Your Home

I would be remiss in not pointing out that the Consumption Concept can be applied to how you live, not just what you eat. I'm not saying we should forgo conveniences in the way we live at home; instead, I just want for us to bring conscientiousness to what resources we use, how we use them, and how we may be affecting them and others around us. Let's take out corporations for a minute and look only at ourselves.

How big would you build your house if you had to source the materials from nature? How much water would you use if you had to haul it from the source? In the same conservationist vein, would you continue to directly or indirectly ingest or use drugs and chemicals knowing that they end up in the waterways through our waste? Would you then continue to take medication for an ailment that can be cured or eased if you do not engage in the behaviour that caused the condition? Knowing that even modern water treatment systems are unable to remove some drugs and chemicals from your tap water, what drugs would you take knowing that your neighbours and children could be drinking their residue?

What chemicals would you use in your household if you knew you were going to eat them somewhere down the line? If you had to source your own cleaners, for instance, would you choose to wash your windows with vinegar, say, instead of turning your basement into a chemistry lab to produce your sci-fi blue window cleaner?

What produce would you eat if you grew it yourself? Food that had toxic chemicals you sprayed on it from your *Breaking Bad* home chemistry lab, making you sick in the process? Or the food that had a few bugs you had to deal with?

When we return to eating real food based on Nature's Principle, we see how it can be applied further in our lives, and how it can benefit ourselves, others, and the planet. The Consumption Concept could also be called Conscious Consumption. If we want to live well and be well on a healthy planet, we will need to learn to live and eat compassionately, conscientiously, and considerately.

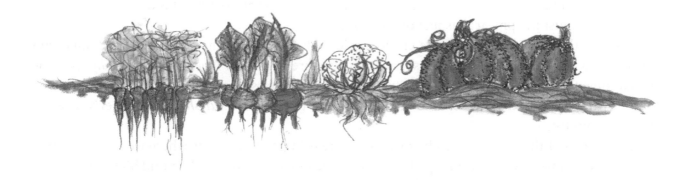

CHAPTER FIVE

HYPERNOURISHMENT

In the *Return to Food* eight-week online program, we focus a great deal on workshopping the concept of HyperNourishment—that is, we look at the intricate relationship between our mental, emotional, physical, and spiritual states. In other words, we examine what it means to be holistic beings.

When one part of our being is out of sync or balance, toxic, or malnourished, it impacts all the other aspects of ourselves. I've observed that when a person starts to remove toxicity in one of the quadrants, their emotions become elevated, and it is much easier, then, to make choices that resonate on a high vibrational level (positive instead of negative) in all the other areas of life.

In this term "HyperNourishment" that I've created, "hyper" does not mean overactive nourishment or excessive nourishment. I use it with liberty in reference to its definition of "existing in more than three dimensions"; in this case, the four quadrants of our human existence. Also applicable is that "hyper" comes from the Greek, meaning 'more than', as our nourishment is dependent on more than food and just the physical aspect of our being.

To look at the four dimensions, we create a grid with four quadrants and divide each quadrant into four, so you have sixteen squares. Each large square is given a label, one being *physical*, one *mental*, one *emotional*, and the last *spiritual*. The four smaller squares in each quadrant are given the following titles: *Malnourished* and *Toxic* in the two top boxes; *Nourished* and HyperNourished in the bottom two.

We then look at the areas in each box where we are bringing in toxicity, where we are not getting enough nourishment, where we are getting nourished, and where we can then find high-vibrational, nourishing things or activities to accelerate our healing and growth.

This tool has been revolutionary in working with clients. It is deceptively simple, yet incredibly powerful when you do it. Your relationship with food heals dramatically faster, because you are working on the underlying behaviours and thought processes that drive the behaviour. Our spirit impacts our thoughts; our thoughts impact our feelings; and our feelings impact our action.

When we do things like watch a horror movie or listen to negative music or read depressing literature, we lower our vibrational resonance. When we're scared or angry or sad, we're not in the best place to make good decisions, because they'll be coming out of our low-vibrational state. The lower our resonance, the less likely we are to seek foods and activities that benefit us. The higher the frequency we have in our body, the more likely we are to choose foods that resonate higher and make us feel better over things made with the Lethal Recipe. Likewise, the more high-vibrational food we eat—refer to Nature's Principle! Living plant foods resonate at a much higher frequency than anything made with the Lethal Recipe—the more likely we are to make good decisions in the other areas of our life.

Below are some examples. It is not an exhaustive list but a start, to give you an idea of what I'm talking about. The sections are not absolute and can carry over into other quadrants.

Examples of Toxic Spirituality

- Being judgmental of others' behaviours in the name of God and religion;
- Rituals of shaming behaviour;
- Demanding others live as you do and believe what you believe.

Examples of Toxic Mental Practices and Influences

- Negative self-talk;
- Watching and reading negative news, crime, violence, horror, and shows in which people complain, perpetuating the victim cycle;
- Reality television;
- Bitching and complaining;
- Worrying;
- Not assuming responsibility where it would be appropriate.

Examples of Toxic Emotional Practices and Influences

- Repeating negative or traumatic events out loud or in "mind movies";
- Addiction to a negative victim mentality;
- Focusing on what's wrong in your life;
- Not forgiving yourself and others;
- Putting others' feelings ahead of yours;
- Bitching and complaining.

Examples of Toxic Physical Practices and Influences

- Eating the Lethal Recipe;
- Being extremely sedentary (going months without exercise);
- Having chemicals in your food, home, cleaning products, and grooming products;
- Excessive electronic and EMF (electric and magnetic field) exposure;
- Staying up late;
- Inconsistent sleep;
- Addiction to drugs, alcohol, sex, or food.

Examples of Malnourished Spiritual Practices

- Not engaging in activities that raise your spirit and connect you with something greater than yourself.

Examples of Malnourished Mental Practices and Influences

- Not reading, listening to, or watching things that help you grow.

Examples of Malnourished Emotional Practices and Influences

- Not asking for what you need emotionally;

- Denying your feelings or making them wrong (this can be toxic as well).

Examples of Malnourished Physical Practices and Influences

- Being sedentary (not exercising daily);
- Eating food that is keeping you alive but not providing sufficient nutrients;
- Not getting out into nature.

Examples of Nourished Spiritual Practices

- Prayer;
- Meditation;
- Yoga;
- Breath work.

Examples of Nourished Mental Practices and Influences

- Positive, inspirational, and high-vibrational input; e.g., books, programs, entertainment.

Examples of Nourished Emotional Practices and Influences

- Time for yourself each day;
- Learning to set boundaries and say no;
- Learning to express your feelings;
- Responsibly communicating how you feel to others.

Examples of Nourished Physical Practices and Influences

- Good food;
- Eating at regular times;
- Regular movement and/or exercise.

Examples of HyperNourished Spiritual Practices

- Prayer, meditation, and yoga for consistent and sustained periods;
- Healing practices;
- Being around enlightened yet humble, kind, and nonjudgmental people;
- Helping others evolve and grow.

Examples of HyperNourished Mental Practices and Influences

- High-level brain engagement through reading, programs, workshops, conversations, problem solving, or brain frequency technologies.

Examples of HyperNourished Emotional Practices and Influences

- Allowing yourself to feel your feelings, move through them, and seek a thought pattern that moves you to a higher vibrational feeling.

Examples of HyperNourished Physical Practices and Influences

- Eating nutrient-dense, seasonal, local, organic, and biodynamically grown whole food;
- Getting out in nature;
- Regenerating out in nature;
- Regular massage, yoga, consistent and sustained exercise, movement, dance.
- Optimal hydration through spring water and high-water-content, living foods.

JORDAN

Jordan, a young, extremely likable executive working in a family business and in demand by headhunters with more job offers and solicitations than he could accept, came to me with his fiancée after struggling with diagnoses of chronic fatigue and glandular fever. Doctors told him he'd need at least eight months to recover and he could be treated only with drugs. His parents, who were corporate clients of mine, asked if I could help.

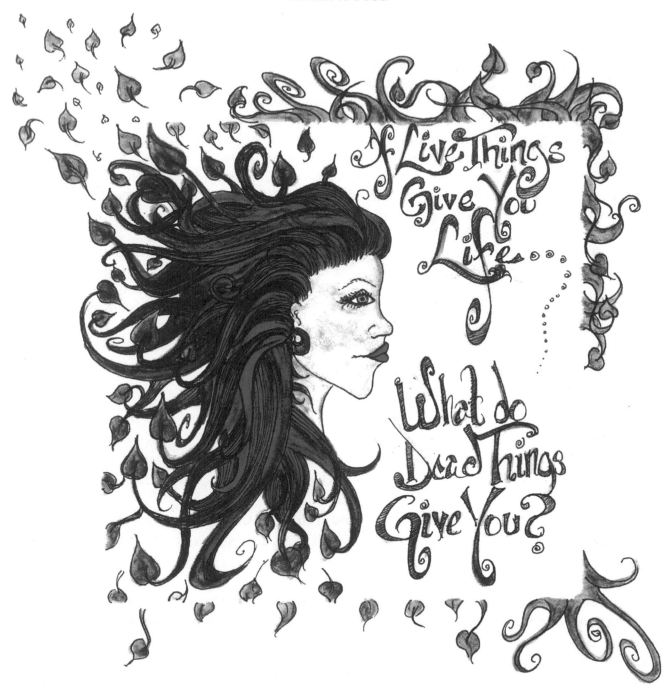

If Live Things Give You Life...

What do Dead Things Give You?

During the health assessment in which I looked at his life holistically, I intuitively asked him if it was easier to get sick than to say no to people. His and Maria's jaws dropped at the same time. The light had come on.

We worked toward him setting boundaries around his work and considering the possibility of following his passions rather than what others wanted and expected of him. We also took three things out of his diet. Within a month, he'd lost twenty-four pounds and reported a 300 percent increase in his energy levels, all without drugs.

The three things we removed were chocolate, coffee, and red wine. Jordan was using these socially acceptable foods as distractions and coping tools to deal with the stress of trying to keep everyone happy. The irony is that his coping tools had the opposite effect: they completely taxed his adrenals and sucked the life force from him.

Often, when we don't have words, we choose foods to soothe and bring us comfort—and rarely is the food a bowl of broccoli or carrots. We choose foods to bring us the drug-like reaction, for example, an increased serotonin level, that represents comfort and soothing for us. The problem is, it creates havoc in our body if the foods are hyper-stimulating or addictive.

Next time you are going through your cupboards or fridge, ask yourself what is there that you may be eating to avoid feeling, and consider what you can replace it with the next time you are shopping. Use Nature's Principle when deciding!

THE MINDSET

"Be kind, for everyone is fighting a battle you know nothing about."
Ian Maclaren

One of the biggest obstacles we face with any kind of change is what's in our head—how we've been conditioned to think, how we condition ourselves to think, and how we approach change through our mindset.

The mind can justify anything.

Think about a time when you wanted something to eat, knew it was not what you needed and in fact was not good for you, yet you came up with a completely logical and justifiable reason to eat it.

I remember craving a cupcake at a busy bakery I loved. I told myself that if there was a parking spot available when I drove by, that would be a sign I could have the cupcake; otherwise I couldn't.

Of course, as chance would have it, the seventh time I drove around the block, there was a space free. See? The mind *can* justify anything.

Be open to the fact that many of your thoughts are not true, which is good, because that means you can change your thoughts for ones that serve you better. Your mind is a garden and your beliefs are the results of the thoughts you plant, water, fertilize, and allow to grow. What are you planting? Noxious weeds, GMOs, organic food, superfoods, medicinals?

Sometimes we just have to get out of our own way. How we think to a large degree determines how we treat ourselves, others, and our planet.

Know that you have genius within you.

Seek wisdom, not just knowledge. You were born with everything you need to know.

Choose the thoughts that serve you and your higher purpose.

Ultimately, what's inside eventually shows up outside. Without starting on the inside, we can never change anything in our physical world for long; the two are intrinsically connected. This is why diets consistently fail—they are working on the external physical behaviour and conditions. Even the best work only for as long as you can sustain them. If your internal language, beliefs, and programming are toxic or malnourished, you will eventually sabotage your diet.

Nourishing thoughts and beliefs are key to creating higher vibrational feelings that lead to healthier actions and behaviours.

The HeartSet

The heart is as complex as the brain. It is not just a pump for our blood; it also carries out complex interactions that impact our gut and brain. According to the HeartMath Institute, your heart emits EMFs that change according to your emotions. Your heart's magnetic field can be measured and felt several feet away from your body. Positive emotions strengthen our immune system, and the heart sends more information to the brain than the brain sends to the heart.

Positive emotions can help you be more creative and innovative, as well as help you solve problems better and make better decisions. When we suppress our emotions, we suppress energy that can become blocked and stored in the body. Sickness, depression, and weight gain can all be tied to suppressing our feelings with food or choosing foods that can actually numb, the way drugs can.

Give yourself permission to feel your feelings, and allow yourself to move through them and feel what comes up for you in the moment. Your feelings are not wrong; they're sign posts to indicate what is happening internally.

Wallowing in your feelings is different from the above, and comes not from not allowing yourself to move through your feelings, but from replaying in your mind thoughts of the past or worries about the future. This cycle often drives us to eat to numb ourselves or escape pain.

Engaging the HeartSet is about choosing the thoughts that produce the feelings that serve our highest good. It is about seeking out the emotions of our true essence, and moving from fear to love.

An integral part of developing a healthy HeartSet is learning to say yes to what you really want, to your higher serving needs, and to what is truly good for your heart, spirit, mind, and body, and no to what you don't want or need and to what is bad for you.

Think back to the HyperNourishment model. You can find physical food that nourishes the heart and physical food that is toxic to the heart; mental food that nourishes the heart and mental food that is toxic to the heart. The same goes for spiritual and emotional food.

Seek a better thought, produce a better feeling.

Addiction Is Never About the Food : A Holistic Perspective

As we learned earlier, food is addictive, particularly if it has been processed. There are powerfully compelling drugs in foods that drive our choices beyond our palates. We can bliss out on them physiologically.

Most people believe that what we choose to eat is based primarily on taste. The truth is, how the food makes us feel drives our choices more. We can develop a palate for anything. Think back to your first taste of coffee, unsweetened chocolate, alcohol, or cigarettes. They tasted bitter, acrid, or astringent, but just as fast as you tasted them and your palate was telling you no, the addictive compounds were already sending signals throughout your body to create a mildly stimulating or drug-like sensation. We subconsciously choose food because of how the food will make us feel while and after we are eating it.

The highs from refined sugar, the serotonin buzz from the tryptophan in meats and certain carbohydrates, and the opiates in dairy all work to drive us to eat more. Chocolate contains a mix of compounds that are compelling or addictive to the body. It can create the same brain compounds as when you are falling in love. These compounds include caffeine, although there is not nearly as much caffeine in chocolate as in coffee, and anandamide, theobromine, phenylethylamine, which create a marijuana-like effect on the brain. When you eat chocolate, your pulse quickens and your body releases the same endorphins your brain produces when you're having sex. These have the potential to raise dopamine and serotonin levels. So it's not just the flavour or sweetness of chocolate that has us going back to it time and time again.

However, addiction is never about the food. It is about how we think and feel. When you get to the root of what you are feeling and the thoughts that propel those emotions, you will understand why you make certain food choices.

When we feel an emotion we are uncomfortable with, the body's natural reaction is to make itself feel better. When we are not practised in training the mind to produce the thought that can make us feel better, we choose a substance or activity to do that instead.

Just as being malnourished physically can drive us to sugar, alcohol, and other addictive substances and behaviours, being malnourished mentally, spiritually, and emotionally can drive us to choose substances or activities to make us feel better, but these are often only short-term surges or highs. The ensuing depletion and lows then make you seek another hit of the "drug."

The nourished mind, heart, and soul tend to make better choices around what they eat, drink, who they do it around, and what stimuli they allow into their sphere. When you are HyperNourished, you will choose books and programs to read and watch that create a sense of genuine well-being and learning. You will opt for food that makes your body feel better, not just while eating it, but long after you have consumed it. A HyperNourished person who is listening to their body will tend to choose to eat appropriate amounts of food, as well, since they are being nourished on the physical, mental, emotional, and spiritual levels.

If you are overeating or choosing addictive substances or activities, consider looking at the various areas of your life that may require nourishment.

PHYSICAL

Observe your food (quantities and quality), water intake, frequency of exercise and stretching, and the quality of your breathing.

Mental

Observe and monitor reading materials, television programs and other entertainment, conversations with others, lectures, and your thought processes.

Emotional

Observe and monitor interactions with others and the thoughts that precede your feelings. Are you able to feel and communicate your feelings responsibly and freely?

Spiritual

Observe and monitor your spiritual activities. Do you have a regular spiritual practice of either prayer or meditation or both? Does your spiritual practice make you feel better for engaging in it or are you left feeling worse about yourself or others? You do not have to believe in God or belong to any religious denomination to have a spiritual practice. It is about engaging the spiritual hardwiring you have within you in a way that allows it to be expressed. There are ways that serve this positively and ways to do this negatively, such as when we do it out of love instead of fear. Obviously, the former contribute to well-being and the latter contribute to being unwell or sick.

Relationship is Relationship is Relationship

There is an expression in the self-help world that "relationship is relationship is relationship," meaning that how you "do" relationships in one area of your life is often how you do them in other areas.

What I have discovered with food is very much along those lines; how you do food is how you do life, and vice versa. If you are fearful, this will show up in how you eat. For years, not unlike others, remembering the scarcity of my childhood, I felt fearful that I would not earn enough to eat well, so when I was in front of an abundant spread of food, I would eat as if I needed to stockpile, just in case it was the last abundant spread I would ever experience. It was also a reflection of the lack-of-abundance mentality with which I struggled on a daily basis.

As you get to know yourself, you will start to recognize these patterns and find that how you do life will show up in ways that you eat and in the choices you make around food. The more you uncover who you are as a person—what truly drives you (not fear or negative emotions)—the more you make decisions in your life based on what it is that you really want in your heart. As you become truer to yourself, you will notice a measurable sense of well-being increase.

Well-being cannot help but increase as you get closer to who you truly are, as well as love and truly accept who you are. The choices you start to make regarding all the aspects that impact your being—including food—will start to be ones that serve your highest good.

Begin to visualize what it is you want from life. Since you're reading this book, chances are you're ready to explore what you can do next to change your life for the better. As you start to spiral up in your energy and thoughts, you will be kinder to yourself.

Take time daily to visualize in this way; dream it, feel it, begin to create it within your mind first.

GUILT, SHAME, AND INGES

I used to say that guilt is completely useless to us when we need to make good decisions about what to eat and how to take care of our bodies; if we felt badly enough, it would be a form of self-flagellation and somehow compensate for our indulgence.

I've since come to learn that guilt performs a useful function in life. Just as the "I'm not good enoughs" (INGEs) do. If there is a universal emotion experienced by humans, you can usually find an evolutionary reason for it. Bestselling author Brené Brown's writing has taught me that guilt is the cognitive dissonance we experience when we've done something that goes against our values. When we hold that behaviour up against our values, it doesn't feel right; we feel guilt.

Thus, there is healthy guilt, the trigger that alerts us of our behaviour and prompts self-correction, and unhealthy guilt, which we use as a tool to punish ourselves into inaction or to perpetuate the cycle of unhealthy behaviour. This kind of guilt can spiral down into shame, which Brené defines as that which corrodes the part of us that believes we can change. Many chronic dieters and people struggling with eating disorders struggle with shame, because in the middle of a repeated unwanted behaviour, it can feel like they'll never be able to break the cycle.

The universal experience of INGEs means that there must be an evolutionary reason for it. I believe it is part of that which drives us to evolve, grow, and want to be better. Just as with guilt, we can use it healthily or we can use it to beat ourselves up, which perpetuates the vicious cycle

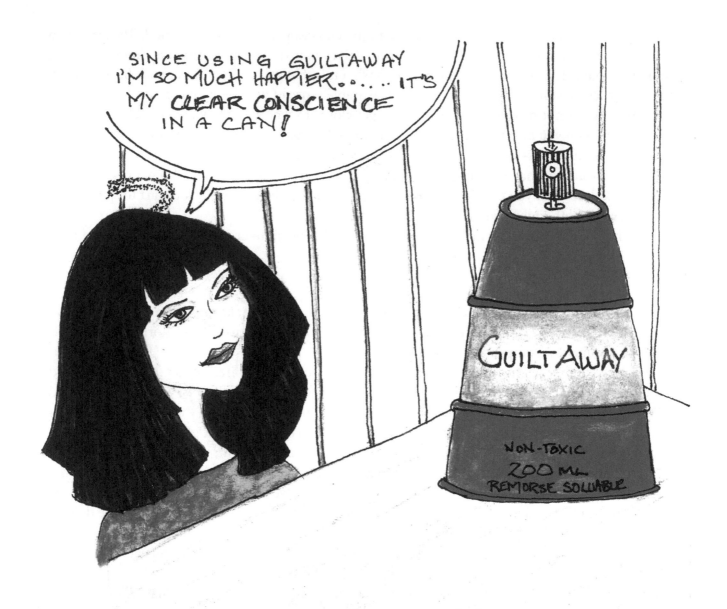

of negativity. When we use it for our personal evolution, we tend to push ourselves to achieve and grow, something that makes us feel alive and brings value to the world.

As a recovering perfectionist, I'm learning to balance my INGEs with "good enough." When I was filming my *Return to Food* online program, I used "good enough" to get it done. Each week, I struggled with releasing it, concerned with whether or not it was good enough. But I consoled myself with the knowledge that I can always go back and make it better. If I'd waited for it to be perfect, it would never have been released. The positive feedback throughout the program blew me away, and though I know there are things I will do to tweak it and make it better, "good enough" was the key to getting the work out there. Years ago, I would have used the INGEs to shrink back. Now, I know that behaviour is actually not a flaw but an evolutionary response that compels me to grow. As I grow within, I use food less as a coping mechanism to deal with discomfort.

The ability for the body to heal is miraculous. In my work with clients, one of the things I encourage is being open to miracles. By all means do the work. And also keep an open mind that each day a miraculous shift in perspective can have transformative effects. I've seen it too many times to believe miracles are for only a chosen few. They usually begin with self-love or simply being open to loving yourself.

Chapter Six

The Universal Recipe for Healing

The physical body has physical needs that are based on laws. The more you work within these laws, the better your body will operate. The mind has the power to override certain laws, but only for so long, and then the body manifests signs of weakness and eventually sickness. When you push the boundaries of nature, something's got to give. Some people with great genetics are able to push things further, but what we are seeing is that the gene pool is weakening as generations continue to eat highly processed food. Some forecast that we now face the potential of a generation of children who will not outlive their parents. For me, that's very sad. It's not natural.

The physical food we feed ourselves is a reflection of where we are mentally, emotionally, and spiritually. Our physical being, what we see, is the manifestation of the unseen.

When you value the body you have been given, are truly grateful for it, and love yourself from a deep, caring altruistic place, it is impossible to consistently feed yourself food that is not designed for it.

There are foods that block feelings of goodness, that mess with our factory settings of happiness, energy, and flow. They are dead foods, foods that have had their natural goodness removed and chemicals added to them, which are not designed for the body. When we eat these foods, it is much more difficult to connect with the body, to find the root causes of ailments in it, and to heal it. It is harder to feel in flow, be happy, naturally energetic, and creative.

Listening to Your Body

Finding peace and developing a healthy relationship with food and your body starts with the ability to hear the constant stream of messages your body is communicating to let you know where you are. With enough highly stimulating and processed foods, your body can reach a level of saturation and actually become desensitized to the messages.

To listen to the body's messages, we need to do two things.

First, let go of the resistance that inevitably comes up as the ego senses change. You will likely have thoughts that this new activity of listening to your body is stupid or not going to help or work, or that you are different from others in some way. Instead of resisting the thoughts, acknowledge them, allow them a voice, thank them very much, and say, "You're welcome to revisit after I practise the next thing we must do."

The second key skill is to get quiet, which is covered after Marie's story below.

For most people, the signal from the body that certain foods are not good for you is not as dramatic as a heart attack or seizures, but the initially subtle messages, if we continue to ignore them, become more intense to get our attention. A cough becomes a cold, a cold becomes a flu, a flu becomes pneumonia, and pneumonia can become lung disease.

In most cases, the signs of sickness from highly processed foods can take weeks, months, or years to manifest to the extremes of disease and death. Also, it is very difficult to trace disease to just one ingredient, one type of extreme processing, or the lack of a specific nutrient. Our bodies are so complex they can manifest toxicity in innumerable ways, making it extremely difficult to assess.

Marie Farugia

A dear friend of mine, Marie Farugia, warns of the dangers of ignoring conditions she describes as "put-up-able"—the things that have you going to a pharmacy time after time. You treat the symptoms and never address the cause, because you don't want to change the behaviour that is causing the symptom. Marie had chronic thrush for years and would take on certain amounts of advice, but only what suited her. She would have a little success with eating well and then, when things improved, she would slip back into the old behaviour that had caused the thrush. It was only when she was diagnosed with cancer that she felt the need to totally clean up what she was eating, address the emotional factors that were creating illness, and change the behaviours that were feeding the cancer.

Three weeks into a juice fast after her breast surgery, she noticed healing in her body and a sensation of well-being unlike she had ever had before. She asked me if the juice fast would have been helpful for her thrush. I said, "Yes."

She asked why I hadn't suggested it, then.

I said, "I did. Twice."

She had a look of disbelief and then self-disappointment. "I honestly didn't hear you," she said.

I said, "Bella, some of us just need louder messages."

Marie now encourages others not to ignore their body's cries to address their health even if the symptoms are "put-up-able" or can be remedied with a pill.

The truth is, sometimes people are more attached to the behaviours, thoughts, and patterns that cause illness. While it is better, of course, to take decisive preventative action that will save a great deal of pain, some people prefer to take that hard route, because they cannot bear to give up their attachment to the default substances, thoughts, and behaviours that lead to the disease.

Get Quiet

There are what seem to be millions of distractions that can keep us from being quiet and listening to our thoughts and the physical impulses of our bodies. Getting quiet, being still, and blocking out distraction is a vital practice in being able to identify the following: hunger, cravings (different from hunger signals), emotional discomfort, pain, physical discomfort, itching, twitching, and even thoughts that are directing us to observe what they may be communicating.

Decoding these messages is another skill we teach at the Return to Food Academy in detail. Getting to know yourself as an integrated being physically, mentally, emotionally, and spiritually is best carried out by the practice of getting quiet, blocking out noise and distractions, and starting the process of enquiry as to what the feelings are telling you. Start to distinguish physical body feelings from emotional feelings and journal about them.

Some of the best ways to quiet yourself so you can pay attention are through meditation, prayer, mindful body scanning, and calming the central nervous system through deep breathing. Any one of these will allow you to get clarity in observing the subtle messages from your body. Consider also listening to meditative or brainwave technologies with your eyes closed, or simply walking in nature.

Plug Into Nature

Nature is our energy source. It is where we find great healing in the form of synergistic foods

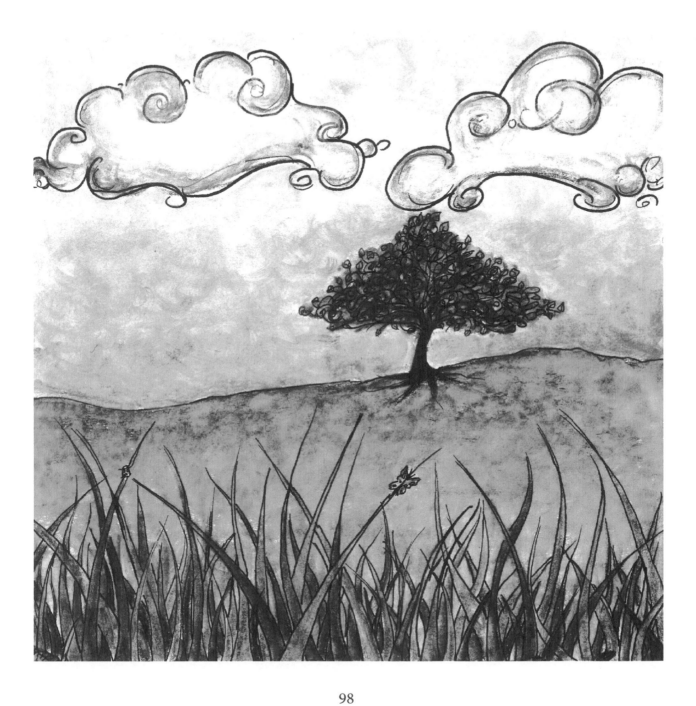

(as close to nature as possible), movement (walking, yoga, swimming), natural environments (parks, oceans, mountains, and nature reserves), silence and calm (meditation, stillness, observing nature, prayer), positive interaction with other beings (therapy, massage, animals, healthy humans), and love and gratitude for ourselves and everything else around us.

The most important thing to keep in mind is that this is your journey; it's unique to you and only you. Take it one step at a time, be patient with your progress, and take it on as a committed new way of doing life.

Some people resonate with keeping written journals, especially when going through change. It could be a great tool for your journey, too. If you already know you like to write, then go ahead: diarize this process of plugging into nature and how it feels from day to day. If you've never journalled, consider this as a thoughtful way to slow down and reflect on what's happening for you as you partake in the various forms of healing.

Though every human is unique, there are ways in which we are all bound by physical laws. Our physical requirements may vary slightly, human to human, but there are elements universal to healing and thriving.

Air

As the most abundant nutrient available to humans, oxygen is essential to every function the body performs, including oxygenating cells and alkalizing the body, which are extremely important for living a healthy, long life. Breathing exercises can calm the autonomic nervous system and reduce stress.

Conversely, a lack of good, clean air can shorten our life span and contribute to the development of disease.

Take in More Air

- Get out in nature for fresh air;
- Practise breathing techniques;
- Exercise; movement increases our oxygen intake.

Air and the Power of the Breath

Breathe in … deeply. Now exhale … deeply. Breathe in again. Now hold your breath for a few seconds … exhale. This breathing we do all day, every day is a vital source of life. Clean air nourishes, cleanses, energizes, and gives life and health to our cells. Despite this, we often overlook air and breathing; we truly take them for granted.

We rush through life, taking short, shallow breaths. We stuff down bites of food while we talk … gasping for air somewhere in between. Stress-triggered eating can be eliminated by being conscious of and practising our breathing. When our bodies are stressed or in a hyper-alert state, our breathing is shallow. Continued states of stress (which have become commonplace today) mean less oxygen reaches our cells, which accelerates the aging process.

Deep, conscious breathing allows oxygen to get to all of our cells, bringing energy and rejuvenation. The more oxygen in our cells, the more healing and less aging or degeneration. One of the reasons athletes are suspected of having lower cancer rates is that as they exercise, they take in regular, deep breaths.

Take the time to consider your breathing. Changing this one, simple aspect of your life, practising slower, more conscious breathing, can improve your well-being in several ways, among which are becoming less stressed, lowering cortisol (stress hormone) levels, and even losing weight.

Water, Hydration, and Your Body

Water is the catalyst for nearly every one of our bodily functions. When our cells are well hydrated, we perform better academically, in sports, at work—in every area of life. Water also lubricates the joints, keep the toxins and other unwanted wastes moving through the gut, and positively affects brain function. In his book *Your Body's Many Cries for Water* (1992), Dr. Fereydoon Batmanghelidj suggests that many diseases could be avoided with the simple act of drinking water and keeping adequately hydrated. He even contends that certain diseases can disappear when you consume healthy water.

Most of society is dehydrated. In fact, an estimated 75 percent of Americans have a drinking problem; they are chronically dehydrated.[13]

If you consider the bioavailability of nutrients as outlined by nature, water is our second most vital nutrient, next to oxygen. Seventy percent of the planet and 70 percent of our body is water, so it makes sense that this should be our primary source of hydration. Most of us know this intuitively, and yet we still struggle to drink the standard eight glasses a day.

Increased consumption of coffee, tea, soft drinks, juices, milk (which is a food not a beverage), and processed drinks distracts people from drinking pure water as their primary source of hydration. Most of these drinks are counterproductive to hydrating the body. As with a lack of oxygen in our cells, a lack of hydration causes us to age quicker, which you can often see evidenced in our skin, which becomes inelastic, papery, and wrinkled when we're dehydrated.

About 2 percent of the water on the planet is fresh, but only 0.3 percent of that 2 percent is usable by humans. Increasingly, less water is clean and suitable for drinking. This is important to remember when you are buying your food and questioning the expense of organics. The basic food stuffs and how they are grown and processed (processing requires the use of water and chemicals) can contribute to either the problem or the solution.

My first memory of drinking water from a natural mountain stream is still striking to me. Travelling through the mountains in Banff National Park on a family trip, my mother insisted we stop to drink water from a fresh stream designated along the road. I remember thinking how odd this was and, in fact, being slightly scared and wondering how this could possibly be good for me. (Another example of our ingrained distrust of nature and what's best for us.)

It tasted sweet, cool, and invigorating.

I now marvel at how one of the most natural experiences was so foreign to this suburban city kid.

Why Are We Drinking Less Water?

If water's so good for us, so refreshing and healing, why are we consuming so little of it? One reason is competition. Billions of dollars are being made with the creation of seductive, feel-good, and addictive drinks that can leave water looking like the frumpy sister at a speed-dating event.

People see water as boring and often forget how powerful it is. We overlook how water can help us not only with the all-important health issues but also with making us more attractive: keeping hydrated is good for clean-smelling breath; supple, responsive skin; a glowing complexion; bright white eyes; less hunger and weight loss; more energy; better sleep; clearer thinking; better digestive flow; and less pillow face. Pillow face occurs when your face keeps the imprint of wrinkles from the

clean air • clean water • clean food • cool climate • rich soils

biodiverse vegetation • abundant animal species

lush rainforests • clean oceans/waterways • vibrant ecology

We don't inherit the earth from our ancestors, We borrow it from our children.

Ancient Proverb

what kind of place are you leaving?

Libra Odd Spot # 56: It is estimated that a plastic container will not decompose for as long as 50000 Years

pillow. It is often a sign of dehydration. To avoid this, drink plenty of water and sleep on your back. One of my food-coaching clients reported losing thirteen pounds just from drinking more water.

Healthy spring water occurs in nature by falling as rain and trickling down the leaves of vegetation, down stems, trunks, and into root systems. From there, it travels through layers of mineralized sediment and rock bed, then into streams where it flows and is energized, mineralized, and cleansed.

But many of us don't have access to spring water straight from nature. Our water falls as rain into reservoirs where it is then shot through pipes and chemically treated at a plant, then thrust through more pipes of inconsistent quality to your taps at home. The debates about fluoridation and chlorination could take up their own books, and are well worth doing your own research about. It will be quite illuminating.

But there are so many more things in the highly treated stuff that comes out of our taps besides water, chlorine, and fluoride. Tap water can taste downright awful. I have found that some bottled waters taste better than most tap water; but nothing touches fresh spring water. You would be amazed at how much more water you (and your children) will drink when it tastes delicious.

The instinct to drink water is hampered by its being overprocessed. I believe that one of the reasons for our resistance to tap water is that our senses are saying there is something not quite right with it. In his book *Power Versus Force* (2002), kinesiologist Dr. David Hawkins reveals the amazing results of over twenty-five years of research on the power humans have to instinctively make decisions about how good something is for us without even touching or tasting it.

Similarly, as I mentioned before, Jeffrey M. Smith's *Seeds of Deception* (2003) gives dozens of examples of animals in domestic, wild, and captive environments refusing genetically modified feed versus conventional feed; obviously, they cannot read the packaging the feed arrives in; therefore, it is truly a blind tasting. The animals are instinctively drawn to the feed that is more natural. I believe that, although we are less conditioned to use our instincts and actually distrust them, for the same reason—that is, instinct—we resist drinking chemically treated water.

That said, with addictive, sugary drinking options, the addictive component overrides our instincts and creates a stronger compulsion to drink something that is not good for us.

Eliminating the use of bottled water, which contributes to environmental problems, is an ecological imperative. In particular, avoid the use of lower-grade plastics that leach xenoestrogens (industrial chemicals found in soft plastics that mimic natural estrogen) into the water. These dangerous chemicals are linked to health problems such as infertility and hormonal imbalances.

The next time you are able to try fresh, clean drinking water, particularly from a mountain spring or glacier-fed source, grab the opportunity. Show your kids and grandkids, and introduce them to a refreshing, life-giving experience they will never forget.

How Much To Drink?

The research is quite conflicted about how much water we should drink daily. Some say as little as one litre; some say three to four litres; and others are recommending up to twelve litres a day for super-detoxifying. So as always, I take it back to Nature's Principle: "Nature tells us what to eat and the quantities to eat it in by how easily it is obtained in nature."

The more processed and chemicalized your diet is, the more water you are going to need to drink to hydrate and flush out toxins. Two litres is achievable for most people. If you are active, exposed to high temperatures, air conditioning, and air travel, you require more. If 90 percent of your food is high in water content, then your body will likely be getting enough hydration for you to start to listen to your body's messages and just top up with spring water. Use your common sense, and look for ways to make drinking water pleasurable.

Some Suggestions for Keeping Hydrated

Eat more fresh, live foods. Lettuce can be as much as 97 percent water, making a salad a great way to hydrate. So is a piece of fruit or any veggie that is alive and fresh.

Try good quality, natural herbal teas or, better yet, make your own. I love infusing fresh slices of ginger, fresh mint, and a few lemon verbena leaves for about three minutes. After you remove them, you'll have one of the best, freshest teas possible.

Drink citron presse first thing in the morning. It sounds lovely in French, but it is really just freshly squeezed lemon juice in some warm spring water. Your liver and intestines will thank you for it.

Sleep

Sleep is crucial to our well-being, especially for regeneration. Nature tells us this with the fact that most of us spend a third of our life doing it and, if you eat well, that will be plenty. Try to survive a month without food. You can do it and live, but you can't survive more than twenty-one days without sleep and live. The world record that is a validated time for staying awake is eleven days.

It turns out there is an art to sleeping well, which primarily involves creating an environment that mimics nature.

The Art of Sleeping Well

- Avoid the Lethal Recipe, especially stimulants and toxins, i.e., coffee, alcohol, large meals, smoking.
- Eat primarily seasonal, organic whole food.
- Take the television out of the bedroom.
- Avoid working in bed.
- Start to slow down before bed. Avoid the news, heavy reading material, and tricky conversations for at least an hour before bed.
- Undertake a meditation ritual or a gratitude practice.
- Remove electrical clocks and devices especially from near your head.
- Create a dark environment.
- Wake with the sun.
- Turn off the phone or keep it in another room altogether.
- Try to get into bed and to wake at consistent hours seven days of the week.
- Fresh air and a cool room helps.
- Exercise.
- Use an organic mattress and linens that are appropriate for your body.

Everybody is different. If your diet is really toxic, it's possible you cannot get enough sleep and, no matter how little or how much you get, you may always feel tired. If your body is overtaxed trying to digest and deal with way too much food out of the context of nature, then the burden of this can force your digestive system to shut down. Some bodies feel the effects of overtaxing in an opposite way and poor diet can induce insomnia.

There are plenty of things you can do to sleep well.

VEGETATION

Plant foods are the most powerful substances for preventing disease. When I first studied phyto-nutrients—then called phytochemicals—just over twelve thousand had been identified. About five years later, tens of thousands more had been discovered. Who knows what we are yet to discover about these amazing and most abundant sources of nourishment.

Vegetation is not only the most protective source of nutrients for people; when grown organically and biodynamically, it has the best return on investment of human and planetary resources environmentally, with the least downside and threat to our well-being. It is the most sustainable, ecologically sound way to feed billions.

There is a global zeitgeist that is increasingly promoting an awareness not just of how powerful vegetables are, but also how delicious and satisfying a plant-based diet can be. I promote a plant-based way of eating and believe that what the world needs most for healing is for us to fall in love with vegetation and make it taste amazing, so it is a joy to eat.

In the last chapter, I offer some amazing plant-based recipes for you to start experimenting with.

MOVEMENT

Any diet that tells you that you don't need to exercise to lose weight is telling the truth. You can sit in your chair and not move, yet—with caloric restriction—lose weight. There are plenty of unhealthy ways to lose weight and this is just one of them. Movement is essential for health and well-being. Without it, the body sends a message to start breaking down; we atrophy and decompose.

What once carried great meaning—natural movement—is now often replaced with "going to the gym." Moving our body was once essential to living and surviving. Expending energy was a given; it happened with everything we did—gathering food and water, farming, tilling the soil, hunting, running from predators, clearing land and building our homes, tending nature, walking to get around. For much of human history, our struggle was to get enough food to do all of that—unlike today, when we struggle to find ways to work off what we eat.

It is important to find ways of moving that bring you meaning and pleasure beyond the superficial reason of looking good; this reason alone often isn't compelling enough incentive. Remind yourself that your body cleanses through movement. Observe the feelings of well-being that rush through your body when you're moving. Pay attention to how your mood elevates and how your central nervous system is calmed by movement. Climb a peak to see the view, dance around a fire or your living room, swim or kayak, run or cycle a trail. Choose forms of movement you resonate with, and focus on how the movement benefits you, rather than thinking of it as a punishment for indulging.

We were made to move. With activity, fatigue melts away, aches and pains lessen, and, as we get our blood circulating, even our minds become more focused and aware. Something as simple as a walk can ease stress and increase your awareness of your body.

"A Little a Lot" Versus "A Lot a Little"

Exercise has never come easily to me. I am a homebody. I can stay for days at a time in my cave, so to speak. I know, however, that I am at my happiest and healthiest when I move my body regularly, particularly out in a natural environment or in a hot yoga class.

The phrase that shifted my expectation and motivated me to get out more often "a little a lot," versus "a lot a little." This worked for me because then exercise wasn't overwhelming anymore. Instead, I built up my movement regime from doable bits to a point at which they became a habit that I look forward to.

When you approach the changes I recommend in this book, take them in small steps, small bite-size pieces, so to speak. Do a little bit often and you'll soon find the changes have become healthy habits you don't even have to think about.

SUNSHINE

The sun nourishes us and is vital for building a healthy body. The sun stimulates vitamin D production in our skin by providing ultraviolet rays. Vitamin D is a nutrient for bone formation, calcium absorption in the gut, and organ system maintenance.

Sun also feels good on the skin and is known to help prevent depression. It releases serotonin in the brain, which can help regulate sleep, our body temperature, and even our sex drive.

The body has a protective mechanism to tell you when you've had too much sun. Your skin turns red and then burns, which is a sign that your skin is cooking. Fresh plant foods contain carotenoids that help protect the skin from cancers. When the body is malnourished, its ability to protect itself from sun exposure diminishes.

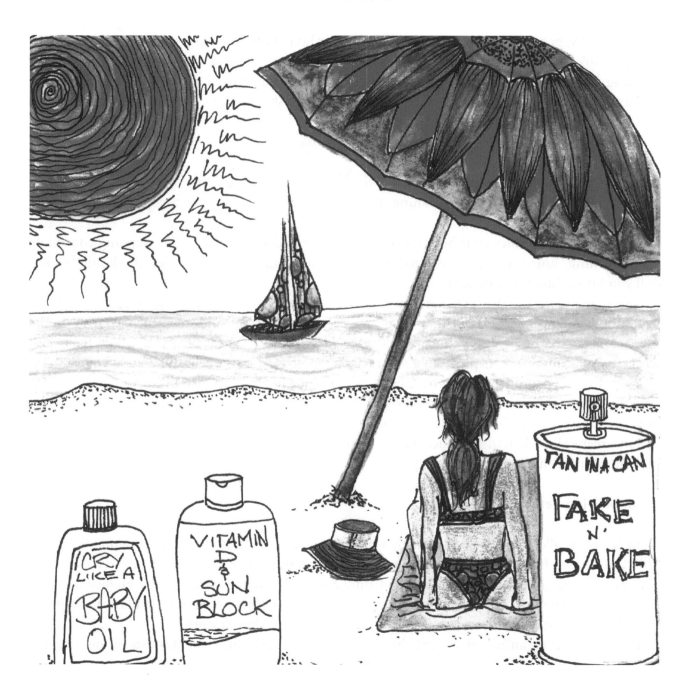

Historically, people did not sunbake on beaches for hours at a time; this concept is relatively new in our history. When traditional healthy cultures were out in the sun, they were usually working, walking, or playing. As I mentioned above, moving the body is healing and protective, and if you do it outside, preferably in nature where the air is clean and fresh, the added benefit is getting sunshine.

The Age of Sunscreen and High Rates of Skin Cancer

Sunscreens introduce chemicals to the body that are so small (through nanotechnology) they enter directly into the bloodstream—meaning they aren't filtered by any protective mechanism in the body.

Sunscreen also disables your body's signal that you've had too much sun. By stopping your body from burning, sunscreens allow you to be out in the sun longer than you naturally should be, and lull you into a false sense of being safe.

If sunscreens were to prevent skin cancer, then it stands to reason that the increased use of them would lower cancer rates.[14] But they do not. In fact, as the use of sunscreen increases, so-do the cancer rates. The best thing you can do to prevent skin cancer is eat plenty of whole fruits and vegetables because of their protective and revitalizing properties for cells. Of course you can also prevent overexposure to the sun by taking note of your body's response to it. It is important to note that the increase of skin cancer directly coincides with the decreased consumption of fresh, organic, raw, properly prepared whole foods.

Sunscreens also block the production of vitamin D, which, as we've established above, is an essential nutrient for the body and cancer prevention.

Sunbathing Versus Sunbaking

Sunbathing is allowing the sun to gently wash over your skin and nourish it. It's done for ten to thirty minutes when the sun is weak, usually in the morning or late afternoon, to avoid strong rays.

Sunbaking is done for longer periods of time and, as the name suggests, the intense heat can actually cook the skin, thereby killing cells. This practice (even with sunscreen that can stop you from burning) should be avoided, especially as it is linked to skin cancers.

There is currently an advertisement circulating that sells the health benefits of sunshine. They tell us it will help us with our metabolism, burn fat, lose weight, and prevent MS, heart disease, and strokes. You'll have better bone health and be in a better mood. Sunshine is good medicine, says the ad, and it's time to rethink the negative messages we are spreading about sunlight. I agree: sunshine is integral to our health.

At the end of the beautiful ad, you discover it was created by the Indoor Tanning Association in America, representing the $2-billion-a-year industry that stands to benefit from you thinking that simulated tanning lights are the same as the light we get from the sun. They are not.

Tanning beds use synthetic sunshine (similar, but not quite the same) and, as with synthetic vitamins and minerals, we are learning that they are not as beneficial for the body. They emit stronger UVB rays than real sunshine; UVB rays give higher levels of radiation.

An August 2014 article in the *Daily Mail Australia* presented research that found that "by the age of 55, people who regularly used a sunbed were 90% more likely to develop SCC than those who did not. Sunbed use was defined as having a 12-minute session about every eight days, or a six minute session every four days, over a 15-year period from age 20 to 35, using a sunbed with a median UV dose. For high dose sunbeds the risk is increased by 180% and even the sunbeds giving the lowest dose found in the 2013 study were linked to a 40% increased risk.[15]"

Once again, we must go back to the principle of this book: when we make choices aligned with Nature's Principle, these problems seem to solve themselves. We choose to be in the sun for smaller amounts of time usually for gardening or exercise; we get out of the sun when our skin begins to burn, indicating that it's becoming damaged; and we wear light clothing to protect ourselves from the hot sun—that is, hats, sunglasses, and light, long-sleeved shirts.

It's all very simple; we've just overcomplicated it. It's important NOT to be afraid of the sun. Just be sun smart.

CHAPTER SEVEN

LOVE, SWEET LOVE AND FOOD, SWEET FOOD

THE MOST IMPORTANT NUTRIENT EVER

The most important nutrient ever is not a new nutrient, but there is a growing global deficiency. It is vital to our growth and the maintenance of life; babies deprived of it die. When this ingredient is added to our food, what we eat not only tastes better, it also feels better. There are no proven food sources of this nutrient; it is generated within us. We can give this nutrient to others and they will flourish, but just as we are weaned from mother's milk to the journey of sustaining ourselves, we need to learn to generate this nutrient within ourselves. If we don't, we will always have a dependency on others for it, which, as with a junkie, will last only until our next hit. As we learn to self-generate this nutrient, we become a more self-actualized individual.

The nutrient is Vitamin L—love. It is not listed in any nutrition textbook as a nutrient we all need, but it is the most significant nutrient for our health, and the fact that we may be deficient, which may be causing our issues, often gets overlooked.

In Chapter Five, I talked about understanding ourselves holistically for optimal health. Learning to observe what the body needs is one thing; learning to observe what the heart, mind, and soul need is equally important. Sometimes the hardest thing to learn is how to self-generate the most nourishing thoughts, the most loving feelings, the kindest actions to propel you toward your true destiny.

What I've discovered with most people who have disordered eating and deficiencies is that there is always a deficit of true self-love. Overeating and eating addictive foods are acts of avoidance. We avoid many things, from difficult conversations with people we love, with whom we want to be but from whom we fear rejection, to even the opposite—difficult conversations with people we are indifferent to but don't want to be with and don't want to hurt. Or we are afraid of the discomfort

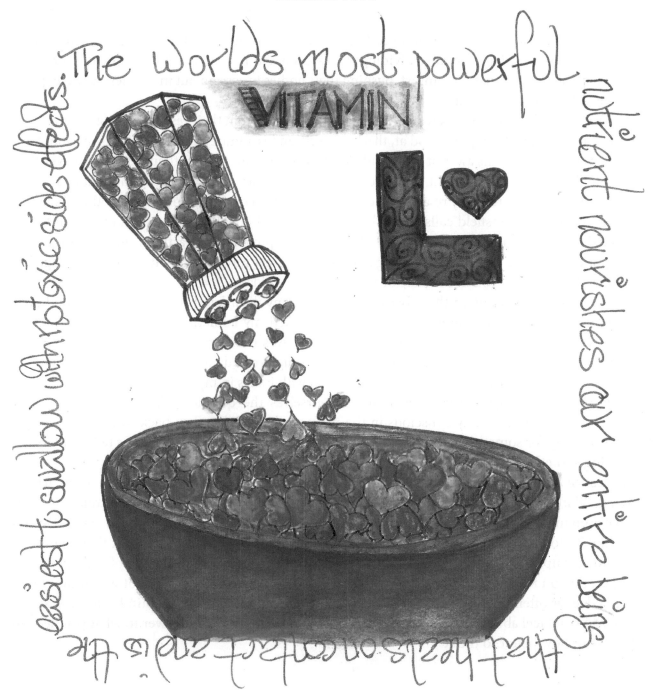

The worlds most powerful VITAMIN L

nutrient nourishes our entire being

that heals on contact and is the easiest to swallow with no toxic side effects.

and change that comes from separation. I know of CEOs of multimillion-dollar companies who stay in loveless marriages because dividing the assets is too hard to conceive. They use food and drink to avoid feeling that discomfort, pushing their bodies to scream out in sickness, a wakeup call they're not yet willing to address.

I've seen people eat and drink to avoid the pain that comes from their resistance to stepping out of the security of the job they are good at, that pays well, and is admired by others. The job is not hard for them to do, but it eats away at their soul. All they really want to do is their art, or whatever they feel called to do. But it is fraught with uncertainty and they are afraid of being thought of as crazy or experiencing failure. They're also reluctant to reject the comfort of the lifestyle their "shadow career" (as Steven Pressfield calls it) has brought them.[16] I know this all too well myself: at first, I pursued my true calling in a half-assed way, not fully stepping into it, fearful of success, as much as I fought even saying those words. Eating bad food is a great way for a nutritionist to sabotage her success. Plus, it keeps you in the state of addiction and avoidance.

I've also been caught up in the process of displacing my disordered relationship with food onto eating healthy versions of food, thinking that I'd kicked my addiction, because I was choosing whole, organic, and raw foods. All I'd done, though, was transfer my wrong thinking to whole versions of the foods through which I'd previously sought avoidance. It was an improvement, an evolution, but not to be confused with fully dealing with issues in my relationship with food.

Our intuition always answers us if we ask ourselves the question, "What am I avoiding?" Sometimes, we are not fully conscious in the moment, but when we go back to the cupboard or fridge looking for something, just a little something, again and again, our action is telling us we are avoiding something.

Unless of course we are truly malnourished—then our body might be sending us to the fridge, saying, "Eat some broccoli." But if we get that message and balk at eating the broccoli, that resistance is giving us a clue as to what's really going on. Examine what's behind your resistance. Do you feel like it's too hard to eat well, with all the food prep? Are you afraid if you start that you might have to give up all the food you like? Do you crave something sweet instead (sign of addiction)? Go deeper: do you feel like you don't deserve to eat well? Do you feel like you're not worth the effort? Going deeper often reveals what we talked about earlier: a deficiency of Vitamin L—love. Examine how you truly feel about needing to eat well and you may just find the answer to what you need to do next or how better to think.

My best tip for long-term weight loss is to "follow your bliss." These famous words of American author Joseph Campbell are some of the purest and wisest words for healthy human behaviour. Avoiding following your bliss should come with a Surgeon General's health warning: "This behaviour will cause weight gain and stress-related problems."

Chances are, we are always avoiding or resisting something as we evolve toward self-actualization; it is part of the journey. It requires courage to self-actualize, and when we do it, it includes some of the most delicious, nourishing acts we can do for ourselves. The best acts for me are getting quiet, meditating, getting out in nature, going for a walk—all acts of self-love, by the way. I ask myself, "What is going on? What do I need? What am I avoiding? How do I act in the most self-loving way right now?"

As my levels of self-love grow, my relationship with food becomes kinder, more loving, and peaceful. It's still a work in progress, but the work is so much more enjoyable with the life-changing anti-diet approach.

What I desire most now in my life is peace. Peace in my relationships with others, myself, and with food. The best way I can think to do this is to fall in love with food, my body, and the planet in the healthiest way possible. When I love the planet, I choose food that is good to the earth, which happens to be good for my body. When I choose food based on loving my body, it's food that happens to be good to the planet. So, I want to proactively develop a deeply loving relationship with food. A healthy kind of love, not an infatuation, even to move beyond my current professional and personal obsession. The irony is that as I heal my relationship with food, I feel compelled to move on and teach other things; I can see the transition occurring now as I teach others to become Return to Food coaches and leaders.

"What the world needs now is love, sweet love" ... and food, real food. If we loved ourselves more, we'd choose more real foods over processed foods. It is the processed, most addictive foods that are causing the most environmental damage; there is a direct connection to our self-love and our love of the planet.

There is a story in First Nations culture about a grandfather and his grandson discussing negative thinking. I feel it's a powerfully relevant parable in relation to this quest of ours to have a healthy relationship with food, our body, and the environment.

The grandson goes to his grandfather feeling there has been a great injustice done to him by a friend. The grandfather tells him there is a battle going on inside each of us, in which two wolves are

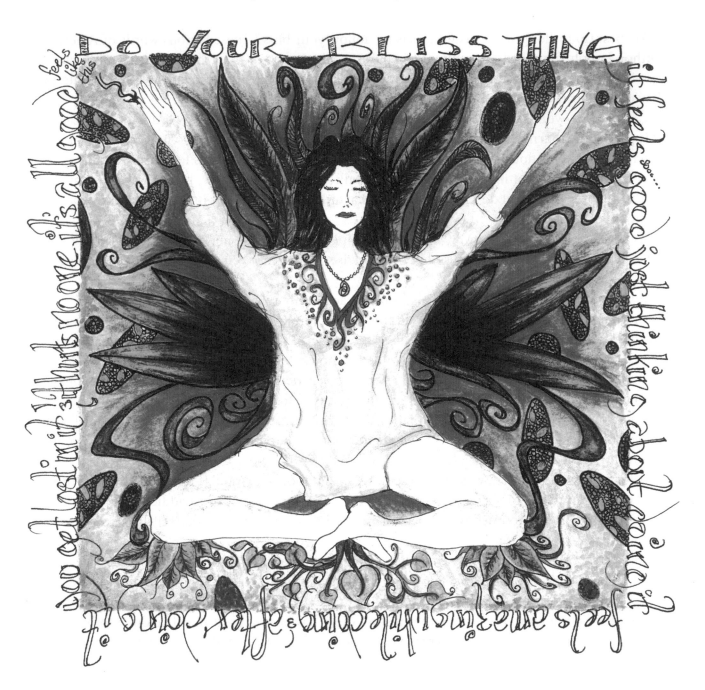

fighting. One wolf is all the bad things within us, like anger, pride, jealousy, regret, envy, self-loathing, lying, and sadness. The other wolf is the good things within us like love, humility, peacefulness, honesty, integrity, generosity, kindness, joy, and truth. Reflecting on his grandfather's words, the grandson asks, "Which wolf will win?"

The grandfather simply replies, "The one you feed."

Seems like a double metaphor for an eating addiction. But as I talked about earlier, what and how we eat in the modern world is rarely about food. For the most part, we eat because of the way it makes us feel, which is often purely physical rather than holistic and reflective of self-love. Sometimes, we feel truly good from the nourishment that comes from food. But more often than not, we confuse the addictive properties in food for sensations of well-being.

It can be tricky to separate the two feelings, as many nourishing foods have addictive properties in them, too. Milk keeps an infant suckling, not just to satisfy hunger and for nourishment, but because of the natural opiates. This is nature's way of ensuring the survival of the infant—by "hooking" it. Nature then moves the child onto other foods by "unhooking" it from milk, by stopping the production of the enzyme lactase that breaks down the lactose in the milk. If a child continues to drink milk beyond weaning, it has to learn to cope with the feeling of discomfort of lactose intolerance by tapping into the feeling that comes from the opiate receptors being tantalized. This is common in our world, as most children are not taught to trust their bodies, but instead are told what they are supposed to eat.

Numerous studies have shown that when given the choice between highly addictive foods and healthy foods, a child that is accustomed to addictive foods will consistently choose the hit from any of the components of the Lethal Recipe over broccoli. Only children who've been trained to trust their bodies or who simply allow themselves to be guided by what makes them feel well will choose the broccoli. Even so, as we know, there is broccoli and then there is broccoli. Eating is no longer a natural process for most of the world.

Our drug receptors are very powerful. Our sugar receptors don't stop at the tip of our tongue as was once believed. They are all over the mouth, the esophagus, and the gut. Which is why it is so unsatisfying to just chew a sweet food and spit out; like foreplay without the climax.

Our food choices helpfully express what's going on in our internal world; they are an outward manifestation of what is occurring in our minds and hearts.

JUDGMENT AND EATING

Not long after I produced and was the presenter in two raw food DVDs (*Seven Recipes for Life* [2009]); *Seven Smoothies for Life* [2010]) I went to a raw food potluck where, in mingling, someone asked me what percentage I was. I looked at her, questioning what she meant by percentage. My sexual orientation, racial mix, or my tax bracket? So I leaned in and asked what she meant.

"What percent raw are you?"

I was taken aback, and said, "Sometimes 5 percent, sometimes 50 percent, some days 90 percent." I shrugged.

She looked at me and said, "You'll get there."

I felt like I'd been "shoulded" on. How yucky.

The more extreme the diet or religion, the more fundamentalist the attitudes people have about others, and the more judgmental, too. There are plenty of vegans, vegetarians, raw foodists, and other natural eaters who live close to their convictions yet don't feel the need to convert, judge, or make others feel bad about their food choices. They are a pleasure to be around. And there are those who see their choices as "the way": anyone who doesn't see the same is doing it wrong, and their health is doomed.

I do a bit of a raw foodist parody in my presentations, where I talk with a bit of a Southern Baptist drawl. "You must not eat that cooked food. That cooked food is the food of the devil. If you eat that cooked food, you're going to be condemned to die a horrible painful death and go straight to hell. What you want is the raw food. The raw food is the way of the Lord and the Light. You eat the raw food and you will be healed; you will be saved; Hallelujah and amen!"

The way people talk about it, it's as though raw food is your only ticket to heaven. For some, eating a raw food diet helped create such a dramatic turnaround in their health that they felt they'd been delivered from hell to heaven. That is their reality. It becomes problematic when they expect others to have the same experience and level of conversion. It is this "zeal of the newly converted" that drives such dramatic movements of people seeking, ensuring sales of products that "will certainly heal you."

Judgment is as toxic to the soul as junk food is to the body. I've said before that I'd rather eat a greasy bowl of noodles with people who are loving, funny, positive, and upbuilding than the most gourmet nutritious meal with people who are angry, passive aggressive, judgmental, negative, or unkind. There is true beauty and power in sharing food that is nourishing, energizing, and protective with people who are kind, loving, and nonjudgmental. That is what the French proverb below epitomizes for me.

Where love sets the table, food tastes its best.

One of the quickest ways to create resistance to this new path toward well-being is judgment of others. It can be so subtle and most people are completely unaware they are doing it. If you find that people are resistant to your new way of embracing food and health, start to look at where you may be judging others. In the *Return to Food* online program, most people insist they don't judge others, and then they do the homework and are surprised by the subtle ways they elevate themselves through judgment. Even if it is nonverbal, people feel it. As soon as people become aware and switch to empathy and compassion, even without saying a word, those who felt resistant, even adversarial, come around.

Telling people what they should and shouldn't eat from a place of judgment is a repellant. When you share from the heart, with joy and gratitude for what you have, where you are, and how amazing all of this real food is, then you make it taste great and you will naturally attract and draw people to it.

Those who are grounded in their beliefs typically do not feel the need to convert others, but are happy to share what has worked for them, to guide and direct without judgment. Those who are not fully rooted in their behaviours are not comfortable with others who do not believe or behave the same or make the same choices. When we are establishing new behaviours, it can be precarious to associate with others who are still engaging in the manners that once made us sick, particularly when we are still struggling with the attachment and detachment ourselves.

Perhaps the harshest judgment to overcome is that from ourselves, we who too often condemn ourselves with every bite and drink misstep or deviation from our desired path. I find that those who are the most judgmental of others are also the hardest on themselves. Being critical of others is often simply a reflection of us rejecting a part of ourselves, the part we fear will lead us away from our new path.

The antidote to all of this is love—love of ourselves and self-loving practices including forgiveness—

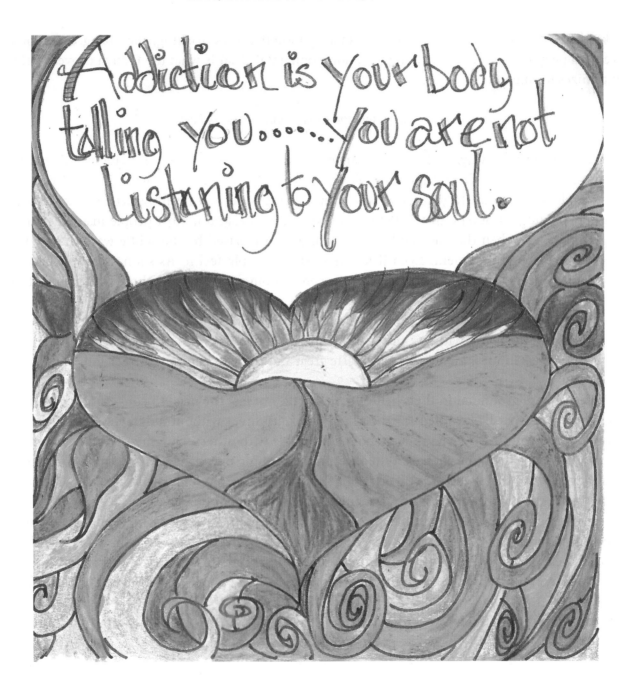

love of others no matter what they believe and do. Sometimes, self-love is separating ourselves for a time from, or at least limiting contact with, temptation. If you are overcoming a serious sugar addiction, perhaps working at an ice cream or candy shop is not the best idea.

Family and partners can be the most sensitive people to navigate. So many triggers go off in the company of those we know intimately or have known over long periods of time. After my weekend-long workshops, I'm often asked by people who are fine when eating alone how they can effectively manage socializing with other people without being made to feel bad or judged. The best way to not be judged is to not judge others and just get on with what you need to do. Just keep it about taking care of yourself and expressing what it is you do and don't feel like doing, not about what you should or should not have. "I really feel like a big bowl of miso soup with tons of veggies" is easier to hear than "I should have a big bowl of miso soup with tons of veggies." Or "You know, I don't really feel like pizza tonight. I find it bloats me and I get heartburn" is easier to hear than "I shouldn't have pizza; it's really bad for you."

CONNECTION AND COMMUNITY

As we move further and further into the technological age, we are tempted to experience life more through technology. Increasingly, we are connecting more superficially—online, through computer games, chat rooms, dating sites, chat windows, quick networking functions, and forums. We have larger networks of friends than we once had, which can all lead to a bizarre form of isolation. We talk, but real connection and depth is lacking, and we as a culture are feeling lonelier than ever, whereas food is really there, always there. One of the causes of overeating is loneliness. How many of us would eat as much as we eat in private if someone we really respected was there to keep us company? The clearer and more honest I am consistently in all my relationships, the less food I eat and the better choices I make.

We are tribal creatures. In primitive times, isolation from the tribe increased the threat of death. Belonging to, being part of, and engaging in community, and connecting with other people (not just animals) is healthy for us; it helps us to evolve and grow, not to mention feel loved, laugh, and share the experience of life together.

Communication is not necessarily connection.

Eating with another person or with people is a gift that has built the strength of bonds of families. It is something I observe in the healthiest, longest living cultures—they eat together. They share meals, meal preparation, and the procurement of the food. They give thanks for the food on the table, the hands that brought it there, and all the sources of nature that provided so bountifully. Loss of life was respected when a meal was consumed. The gravity of a life taken tempered the voracity of the body's strong physiological desires or blood thirst.

Thousands of meals each day now are consumed in cars, in front of televisions or computer screens, over the counter or the sink, standing up. Less and less are we with those we care about. Mobile phones and tablets, even in the company of people physically with us, constantly distract us and keep us from being fully present, exacerbating loneliness. Even food can be a distraction: there is a difference between food as a conduit of true connection (breaking bread together and sharing a meal), and food being a tool to avoid being completely in the moment. Sometimes, we eat to avoid feeling alone with someone or to avoid really being with someone. The difference is subtle but in both cases can contribute to feelings of satiety and satisfaction. But those are short-lived.

There are plenty of people whose lives would be enriched by the simple act of being invited to eat a meal with you. If you know how to cook, offer to cook. If you don't and you know some-one who does, offer to bring the ingredients and ask them to teach you. Even when someone has cooked food that was pretty close to the Lethal Recipe, I have been so touched by their earnest gesture of reciprocity that it has nourished me on a level that transcends the body. Eating together is very important in the Return to Food approach; it's going back and finding our way forward.

"Do not let what you cannot do interfere with what you can do."
John Wooden

The aspect of bringing love to the table is my favourite thing about this whole process. I love getting my food particularly from the people who've actually grown it. I love unpacking it into my fridge and feeling the joy from a fridge full of lovely things from the market. I love the process of deciding what things I'm going to prepare, particularly on the first day of the farmers' market. But on the days when ingredients thin out, there is an equal delight in the challenge of how creative and clever I can be with less and less. Even after all these years in the kitchen, I am always surprised how little it takes to make something delicious when I start out with quality ingredients.

Sharing all of this with people will change your life. The process of returning to food is made infinitely easier by being around like-minded people who are also interested and passionate about real food. You can connect and share resources, recipes, and places to shop; have cooking bees; go on visits to farmers' markets and gardens; and of course, create and share meals together.

If you don't have a community around you, and your family is not yet supportive, you can start online or find people locally who are interested in starting a community. Check out the Return to Food Facebook page (www.facebook.com/returntofoodtv), where you'll find all kinds of people who are interested in the concepts and philosophies in this book. It is a loving, supportive community of people who are passionate about food that nourishes, energizes, and protects body, spirit, mind, and soul.

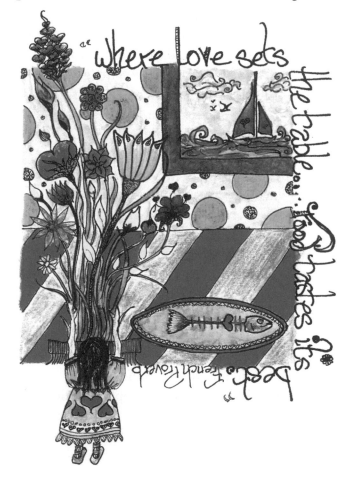

We Are Meant to Eat Together

Eat with people whom you love and respect, who love and respect you,
and who love and respect food.
Eat with people who are learning to cook, with sincerity of heart;
children are a great example of this.
Eat with all your senses, masticating textures, smelling sensuous aromas,
tasting luscious flavours.
Eat with people who aren't afraid to make noises like
ummm, ahhh, and oohh.
Eat with people who aren't afraid to make a mess, lick their fingers,
clean out the bowl, and eat with their hands.
Eat after the perspiration of a rigorous jog, invigorating walk, in the
lusty afterglow from a roll in the hay; it's much healthier than smoking a
cigarette.
Eat with people who laugh and smile a lot,
people who tell stories and spin yarns.
Eat with people who are generous and share. Full stop.
Eat with all your fondest memories, triumphs through tragedy,
and memories of love.
Eat with people who love to cook and eat.
Eat with people who are gracious and grateful.
Eat with people who are nonjudgmental and forgiving, who can see both
sides of the story and still have an opinion.
Eat with love, passion, compassion in your heart,
and while searching your soul.
Eat with people who love life and are genuinely interested in you
and the world around you.
And finally, if you eat like this and with people who do and are all these
things, pleeease … invite me for dinner.

Years ago, when I was coaching the police force in Australia, I had a woman with aggressive body language ask me, "Yeah. Well, how do I get all these happy, loving people to have lunch with me?"

I replied as gently and kindly as I could, "You become one."

Not so many years before that, I was a grumpy, angry person who ate a lot of meals alone. I ate in front of the television, at the sink, or in my car. I ate way more than I would have had I been with loving company. It's not just about the watchful eyes of others; it's about the connections we make, about sharing conversation, challenges, and our victories, no matter how small or great. As humans, we require a sense of community, sharing, and caring that gives us an inner strength that we then use to make better, more nourishing food choices.

Today, invite someone to share a meal with you and remember to show up at that meal as the person you'd like to dine with.

A Note on Eating Mindfully

Whether you are with people or are alone, there are also many advantages of eating a meal mindfully in silence, being aware of each bite and what the food and your relationship with that food brings up. This is a powerful step in healing your relationship with food. As an active exercise of reflection, when done consistently, eating mindfully will create a powerful connection between the intelligences in the food and in your body. In our world today, our lifestyles, eating habits, and most processed food encourage the opposite of connection. This disconnection from our own intelligence leads to our eating foods that aren't good for us, to eating larger amounts of all foods including healthy ones, and to disconnecting from nature; all of these contribute to disordered eating.

Touch as Nourishment

Humans are extremely sensitive to touch. Providing it is good and not violent, touch is so powerful that a newborn can die in the absence of it. Touch is a visceral communication of energy, so it is vital we give and seek out touch that is as nourishing as organic whole food.

Living in a world of virtual friendships and virtual business, we can actually be starved of touch. It is vital to find ways to bring that into or back into your life.

Hugs

Through a reconnection with family and friends, make an effort to give genuine hugs that will make you actually feel the transference of energy. Set the intention of giving love without expectation. The act of giving touch is as powerful as receiving it.

Massage

Find a healing massage therapist and invest in healing touch. Know that it may take time and experimentation to find the therapist who feels right for you.

Two-Handed Handshake

When someone goes to shake your hand, gently—with simple kindness and the intention to connect—place your left hand on top of the other person's hand, look them in the eyes, and notice the difference it makes with people.

Animals

A pet can be an incredible source of love, affection, and satisfying connection. The ability and capacity an animal has to love and connect is in many cases greater than ours. They can provide affection no matter what you look like, feel like, think, and feel about yourself, and no matter how well you've performed at work or what you've done in the past. And they will do this with species other than their own, besides humans. They are amazing beings to practise healthy touch with, both giving and receiving.

This is a short list, but you will be amazed by how healing pleasurable touch is to the body and soul, and how this can translate to healing and vitality.

FINDING YOUR PATH

Knowing yourself is vital to making any change. Be honest. Look back at times in your life when you were successful at making a change or accomplishing a goal. What did you do that worked? What did you do that didn't work?

Look at what you perceive as failures too—also called "learning prep work." What didn't work there? What did work?

It doesn't matter how anyone else is living and making changes. There is no need to pass judgment on yourself (or others) with this honest look. Where you are is simply where you are. Don't fall into the trap of comparisons; that's a recipe for misery. Understand what works for you, embrace it, and get started. This is your journey and no one else's.

I love the parable of the tortoise and the hare: the moral is that slow and steady tends to trump fast and complacent. The best way to see this Holistic Hero's Journey you're on is as a race with a series of finish lines that—if you just keep going—you are going to cross. The weight-loss industry is all about the hare. Ten pounds lost in ten days. It is part of the quick fix, but it rarely encourages work on the inner stuff that drives long-term change.

Know Yourself First

"This above all: to thine own self be true."
William Shakespeare

Part of making changes is how you adapt. Are you a fast or slow adaptor? This is vital to know about yourself to help with any kind of change. Some high-achieving type As convert overnight; others, like me, take a long time to make changes that stick. It's good to note how you develop understanding and patience.

I've rarely met a fundamentalist that was fun to be with,
but quite a few that were mental.

It is all or nothing for fundamentalists, and they basically do a 180° turnaround overnight. I've observed people who become almost religious in their new approach to food and cannot understand why everyone else does not "see the light," come along, and switch as quickly as they have.

If this is not the way you do things—if you are a slow adaptor like me—but you want to live the *Return to Food* approach even though it's not in your nature, you may find it difficult to maintain.

Unless you have a massive incentive to make dramatic changes, like a serious or life-threatening health condition or chronic pain, you may find yourself slipping back into old patterns and then being critical of yourself. You may think that this new way of eating and living is just not for you.

Knowing yourself and how you are most likely to succeed will help you to make changes successfully. Think of the tortoise and the hare. Both can achieve success with the right attitude. Know who you are and how you are most likely to cross the finish line of the goal you set for yourself.

The key is to determine your own innate way and follow that path.

CREATIVITY

We are creative selves. The capping of our creativity is toxic to our whole being. Almost every client who has come to see me with illness or excess weight gain has capped or limited their innate desire to be creative in the way of their gifts and soul's direction.

Expressing your creativity will unblock energy that could be generating a negative vibrational ebb in your body and leading you to eat foods that vibrate at a lower resonance. It is a myth that you need substances outside yourself to trigger creativity, though eating might be an access path for some. They use it as a crutch to lower their resistance to allowing the creative flow to come through them.

The truth is, not creating is unnatural for us. We all possess the ability to create because we were made to do it. But we lose touch with that ability when we don't pay attention to ourselves and our desires. We're residing in an unnatural state. And if there's anything we've learned in this book so far, it's that unnatural doesn't serve us. It's not being true to who we're meant to be. So when we don't create, we become miserable, even depressed. When we don't eat as nature intended, we feel sick and become unwell. In both cases, we are not in a state to make good decisions for ourselves.

One way I look at creativity is that it comes *through* you, more so than coming from *within* you. It is almost as if the ideas that you allow to move through you into your creative outlet act as a cleansing, in the same way that movement cleanses the physical body. Creativity keeps energy flowing. When I've created something, I feel energetically like I've had a great workout.

Observe where you are drawn to express your creativity, no matter where or how your intuition calls you to be creative. It can be in the kitchen, with numbers, art, science, literature, exploring a path of learning and experimentation, or in music. There is no end to the possibilities, and if you think there is, you definitely need to get creative.

Pleasure and Fun

"It's when pleasure ends that overeating begins."
Geneen Roth

Finding joy, pleasure, and fun in every day is a prescription I give my clients and students. This is definitely a "teaching what you most need to learn" aspect of my life that I'm working on. Find the pleasure in everything you do and I promise you, healing and weight loss will ensue.

Pleasure is universal to the human experience—at least the capacity for it is, though what gives us pleasure differs for each of us. When we learn to truly love and HyperNourish ourselves, and then listen to our body, express our creativity, stop using guilt as a tool for self-flagellation, and respect the messages that are coming forth, there is this fabulous transformation that happens. We start to crave foods that actually nourish us, foods full of intelligence, nutrients, and living energy. When we give ourselves permission to experience pleasure and express our highest purpose, we tend to choose foods that also serve a higher purpose. When we block or restrict our healthy human desires, we tend to choose foods that help us suppress the negative feelings that our behaviour creates.

A part of the coaching work I do that I absolutely love is helping people discover their life's purpose and its unique expression.

Jena LaFlamme is the author of *The Secrets of Pleasurable Weight Loss: The Stress-Free, Guilt-Free Path to Loving Your Body and Feeling Great Losing Weight, and Loving Your Life Today* (2015). She has a fabulous take on how our bodies are like loyal, loving dogs that are also amazingly forgiving. She says this about our bodies: "They give us warning signs—that's what weight gain is. Weight is your body's cry for attention, a cry for help. If you're overweight, you can guarantee your body tried to let you know in subtler ways that it wasn't getting its needs met, and eventually it resorted to weight gain. It's like, 'Hey, the way you are eating and living is not working for me. You didn't notice the bloating. You didn't notice the constipation. You didn't notice the rash. Alright, here, try 20 pounds, or try 200 pounds in your case. Are you going to notice me now? Hello!'"

There is a wonderful interview with Jena at www.returntofood.com/jenalaflamme

Discipline and Pleasure

I never liked the word "discipline." I used to associate it with deprivation, hard work, and punishment. Then I found author David Campbell's quote, "Discipline is remembering what you want." When I learned that by focusing deeply on what it is I truly desire, and that discipline is the vehicle that could get me there, my relationship with discipline transformed.

One of the issues is knowing what you really want. When you're reaching for a goal outside of you that isn't truly what you want or that's not connected to your purpose, it's easy to lose focus. When you are deeply connected to your purpose and you acknowledge what you have to do to get there, the hard work, and the hurdles that will inevitably come up, you handle everything from a different perspective—it all feels different from how it feels when you do things for reasons that are not true to who you are.

Imagine you have to move heavy rocks and tons of soil by hand because you're in prison working off a debt to society. How does that feel? Contrast that to moving heavy rocks and tons of soil by hand because you are creating a lovely landscaped garden with the most beautiful plants you can imagine. Pursuing a goal mindful of the beautiful outcome has a totally different feeling than "having to."

Finding Purpose, Meaning, and Contribution

"When we quit thinking primarily of ourselves and our own self-preservation, we undergo a truly heroic transformation of consciousness."
Joseph Campbell

Clients are often challenged by identifying their purpose, meaning, and contribution. They wonder what those have to do with what they eat and with developing a healthy relationship with food, their body, and the planet.

It has been my experience that most people who suffer from a lifestyle-related sickness also suffer from ignoring their soul's calling. They've put their hopes, dreams, and aspirations aside to pursue more practical things like making a living, buying a house, and doing what they should do, instead of doing what their heart is truly calling them to do. I'm not suggesting people abandon their responsibilities and commitments. As I suggested before, you can always find a way to follow your bliss, even if it is for only a few moments each day.

Working together, my clients and I start to excavate their dreams and desires, and implement plans and strategies to start incorporating their heart and soul's calling into their life. Then, miracles happen around their relationship with food.

Aim to find out what it is that lights you up and you will be starting a very important part of nourishing your soul. You'll find that it will also help you in nourishing other parts of your life and body.

We're all here for a particular reason. Some of us, in fact many of us, have lost sight of that as we trudge through our daily lives feeling tired, fatigued, stressed, going to jobs we hate, and living on a schedule that involves little play and even less spirituality.

It's vital to become aware of what makes you happy. What makes you shine? Is it hiking, sewing, the outdoors, travelling, reading, drawing, cooking? When we were babies and young children, we were innately drawn to certain activities, ones that we were made for.

If you've lost that knowledge, take some time to rekindle it. Explore life again, discover yourself. When you couple this with soulful, natural, healthy eating, all will fall beautifully into place. You really can't have one without the other. It's all connected, just as we're all connected.

Do this for yourself, your loved ones, and really, the world. Learn to love life again. If you haven't lost this connection, continue to nurture it in yourself and those around you. Purpose comes from within you. Find what it is you are so good at and use it to help others. Ask yourself what you would be doing if nothing were holding you back.

Pastor and author of *The Purpose Driven Life* (2002) Rick Warren talks of using what is "in your hand"—meaning, your unique abilities, skills, talents, and resources—as your sphere of influence, power, and gifts to serve others. Oprah often prays, "God, use my life for something bigger than myself."

Many successfully recovering alcoholics and drug addicts say one daily prayer to help centre and ground them. Part of this prayer says, "God, I offer myself to you—to build with me and do with me what you will…. May I do your will always." I often use this prayer and the prayer I learned from Oprah to ask for my life to be used for something greater than myself, greater than I know. Then I get to work each day to explore this.

Following the course you were made for—that nature has in store just for you—keeps you in the flow of life, and therefore happy. When you discover what it is you are passionate about and use that to help others, your sense of well-being and self-esteem will rise exponentially. What I find is that when we feel good about ourselves, we are more inclined to feed our body good food, because we do not need to use the drugs in processed foods to make us feel good. Also when we are using our time engaged in service to others meaningfully and powerfully (not as martyrs or victims), we are less likely to be sitting down alone eating food that does not serve us.

Do What You Can One Thing at a Time

A helpful way to think is "this is how I do life" versus "if I can just do this until …" Replace the ellipses with your goal; maybe it's your wedding, school reunion, fortieth birthday, or retirement.

The diet mentality has people walking a tightrope of abstinence until they reach a goal weight. Then what do you do? Most people go back to how they lived before. They eat the foods they deprived themselves of, and in most instances gain back the weight they lost and often even more. In a study by psychologists Traci Mann and Janet Tomiyama at UCLA, dieters actually gained more weight than non-dieters.[17]

The anti-diet approach is all about the belief "This is how I do life." It incorporates life-affirming sustainable changes. Change your life to a higher vibration and the food choices will follow. As you adopt a new positive behaviour and it becomes natural, then you look to change, replace, and adapt even more of your behaviour. So the process is quite natural and organic.

There are different reasons why we make individual choices. I have great respect for the process of making decisions based out of love and not fear. The body will not thrive in an environment of fear; it will heal faster in an environment of love. Most health and weight-loss products are sold very much around fear-based philosophies, because they make people buy faster. Fear is a powerful motivator. But many of these products are like the stones in the stone soup fable—catalysts to attract people to give what is wanted. You already have the most important ingredients. Use them.

My suggestion is that you create a very personal to-do list. Tackle what you can and approach that which is most important with a long-term strategy and positive mantra: "No matter what the setbacks are, I will continue on the course to be drawn to that which heals me, and avoid that which causes me harm." Your to-do list will evolve and change as a result. In time, you will think back to when contemplating making such a change was so big and scary, and you'll smile as you see how, now, it is how you "do" life. You just have to start.

SOURCING OUR FOOD

We've gotten so far away from sourcing and preparing homemade, healthy meals that many people don't even know what it would mean to do this. They wouldn't know where to begin. That's okay. Wherever you are on this journey, accept it. If you're ready to start thinking a bit differently about it, let the words on these pages guide you.

What I mean when I say "source our food" is to shop for it or gather it. Whether it be in your backyard garden, at your local farmers' market, or the grocery store. Sourcing your food means gathering it for preparation.

When we source (shop for) our food in local, healthy places, it may take longer to gather the items. This may also be true about preparing them for meals. Eating this way, the way that will lead you to health and vitality, will take more time than simply popping a meal in the microwave. But I promise you, it will be well worth it. The key is to be truly present, or mindful, in each of the activities—shopping, preparing, creating, eating. Try to approach each with love, appreciating how you and perhaps others will benefit from the meal. When you make each activity enjoyable and sacred, your entire being profits.

It's important to understand what a homemade meal truly is. Many people mistakenly think that when they choose a box of pasta and a jar of sauce, mix it, cook it, and eat it, they're eating a healthy, home-cooked meal. But essentially, this is a highly processed meal.

The point here is that this pasta and sauce meal can be made as a true homemade delight with just a few extra minutes. Making minimal changes in sourcing and preparing this meal is easy and affordable, and will deliver significant quantities of bountiful nutrients to your body.

I'll guide you later on in this book through pain-free ways to make some of these adjustments.

FINDING MEANING IN A SIMPLE MEAL

Many of us assume that food preparation is a great place to cut down on time. We're used to going fast and sometimes it's hard to change. But when you keep in mind that taking just a little more time for meal preparation will bring huge rewards in all aspects of life—physical well-being, mental health, energy levels, weight, and much more—it isn't so difficult to swallow.

Let's go back to the example of the pasta and sauce meal. Instead of choosing white enriched pasta, select a whole grain, organic pasta, or, even better, Zuudles, which are raw zucchini noodles made with a ZuudleMaker.[18] Rather than using a jar of preservative-laden sauce, pick up a few ripe tomatoes at the local farmers' market. Cut up those tomatoes; mix in some basil, garlic, sea salt, and pepper; drizzle in cold-pressed organic olive oil, and sauté. When finished, ladle the sauce over your cooked noodles (or your Zuudles), and there you have a simple, healthy meal that's taken only minutes longer to prepare, is loaded with vitamins, minerals, and other vital nutrients, and produces less waste.

It really can be that simple. The uncomplicated acts of growing your own herbs and tomatoes (which can even be done in a city apartment) and preparing your own sauces are economical, healthy, and great choices for the environment. We forget how simple it is, because we are disconnected from nature, the source of all nourishment.

THE REPLACE PRINCIPLE

When starting to listen to your body and transitioning to what really nourishes you, there will be a period during which you may have food memories that draw you back to the Lethal Recipe. The Replace Principle is about not denying your desire for a food that may not be nourishing. Until you get adept at reading your body's signals, you can upgrade the foods in which you formerly used to indulge.

If you feel like a sweet treat, select the most natural option you can find, starting with raw fruit and then looking to dried fruit. My Raw Chocolate Slice recipe (made from raw nuts, seeds, fruit, and raw cacao, giving it more nutrients) was my way of weaning off sugar. It gave me the sweet hit I craved without the big low from chocolate that contained refined sugar.

I started out slowly. First, I replaced the commercial ice cream with artisan handmade ice cream, which was far better quality and came in smaller tubs. It took less to satisfy me and cost more, so my consumption decreased. Then I moved to organic ice cream, and later found Coconut Bliss ice cream, which is dairy-, soy- and gluten-free, made with coconut milk, and comes in a variety of flavours. It was the first time I found a truly satisfying nondairy ice cream. Now I freeze fruit for delicious fruit sorbets to blend up in my Vitamix, without added sugar.

Replacing and Upgrading Tips

There are tons of ways to upgrade your present way of eating. Here are some ideas for how to take where you are and choose a better solution.

- Conventional anything to organic versions;
- Organic versions to biodynamic versions;
- Instant coffee or coffee capsules in plastic to organic coffee;
- Organic coffee to roasted dandelion root tea;
- Conventional milk to organic milk;
- Organic milk to homemade nut or seed milks;
- Artificial sweeteners to sugar;
- Sugar to coconut palm sugar, dehydrated cane juice, or raw honey;
- Sugar in baking to fruit or dried fruit;
- Soda water to natural sparkling mineral water;
- Tap water to spring water;
- Confection chocolate to organic handcrafted raw chocolate;
- Choose a natural place versus a drive-through for a burger;
- Choose a lettuce bun instead of a bread bun;
- Graduate from meat burgers to whole food veggie burgers;
- Soy-based vegetarian burgers to whole food veggie burgers;
- Conventional wine to organic and biodynamic wines;
- Alcohol anything to funky, blended alcohol-free creations.

Start where you are and, next time you're shopping or planning, upgrade. With the Replace Principle, you want find the more natural option in keeping with and evolving in the direction of Nature's Principle and the Consumption Concept.

Accentuate the Positive, Eliminate the Negative

Never underestimate the power that limiting time with energy suckers (extremely sarcastic, angry, negative, blaming people) can have on your life.

People who don't accept responsibility for their lives can be debilitating to your health. I know this well, because I used to be one. At least I'm in remission.

Looking at that list of negative people, I can see myself in every one of those traits and understand why, at certain times in my life, friends drifted away.

Eliminating exposure to these people and spending more time with those who have a much more empowered spin on life is integral to becoming a holistically healthy person.

You can associate with people who vibrate at a higher level through the books they write, the speeches they give, and by attending courses with like-minded people. Seek them out in your community by frequenting places you value, like your farmers' market. You can lift up others in your life by example; it is, in fact, the most powerful way to influence and attract people— by doing, not telling.

Toxic or Nourishing Entertainment

The American band Red Hot Chili Peppers tout these words in their song "Throw Away Your Television": "Throw away your television / Time to make this clean decision…. / It's a repeat of a story told / It's a repeat and it's getting old."

How true these words are. The TV seems to repeat the same stories on the news daily, most of them negative and thwarted. As research professor, author, and public speaker Brené Brown says, the news is about what's wrong with the world and who's to blame. The popular, prime time TV shows eerily are variations of the same "news," loaded with drama, violence, and negativity that can zap your immune system. All the while, they're selling you food that isn't good for you or the planet, then drugs to help you with the symptoms that the food has created, or worse, drugs that decrease your discomfort so you can eat more of those foods.

When I began to realize what a negative influence television and the news was on my life, I banished the TV to my garage. Later, when it stopped working, I didn't replace it. What I noticed soon after was that I was lighter; I felt less negativity, worry, and envy, and had so much more time to think about or do things that really matter. That still holds true.

Now, as a former serious TV addict, I occasionally long to flick on the remote, especially when I'm uncomfortable and want to distract myself. What I find is that peaceful activities and thought processes help me deal with those feelings of discomfort, rather than distract me from them. I'll search for inspirational or funny videos online instead.

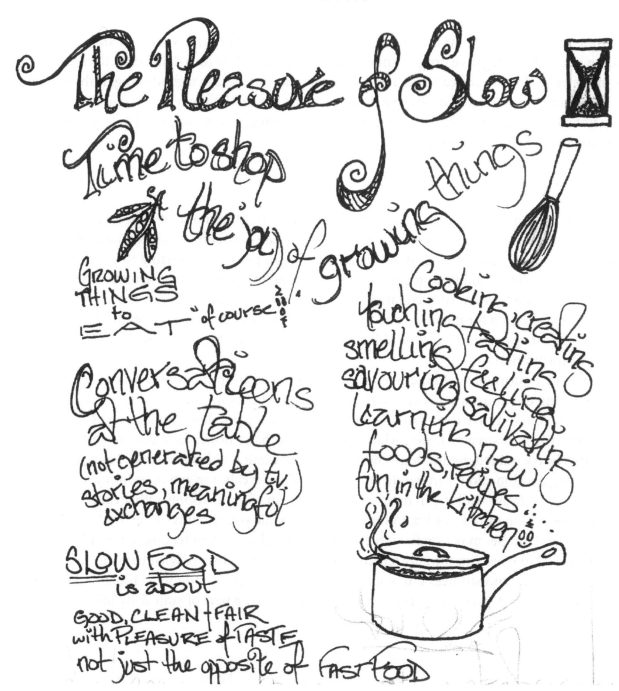

The Pleasure of Slow

Time to shop & the joy of growing things

GROWING THINGS to EAT "of course"

Conversations at the table (not generated by t.v.) stories, meaningful exchanges

Cooking, creating, touching, tasting, smelling, feeling, savouring, salivating, learning new foods, recipes, fun in the kitchen!!

SLOW FOOD is about GOOD, CLEAN & FAIR with PLEASURE & TASTE not just the opposite of FAST FOOD

If your attachment to television is not an issue, then at least observe what you are watching and limit the amount of negative programming you expose yourself to on a daily basis. Reconsider even documentaries that are educational and justified by your intellect as a good thing. If the content of the documentaries is negative, observe the impact that has on the way you feel and think.

I'm not suggesting a head-in-the-sand approach, but you would be surprised to learn how little of what you really need to know is on television.

CREATING PEACE AND STILLNESS IN YOUR LIFE

In modern Western living, it is possible to fill up every waking moment with stimulation in the form of noise, music, ideas, entertainment, food, pleasure—essentially distractions of every sort. We have become accustomed to overstimulation, though people are starting to realize how detrimental this is to their ability to focus and de-stress, and many people are actually uncomfortable with stillness. The thought of meditation and being quiet and still is difficult, even though it is a source of rejuvenation for the mind and body. Healthy cultures in nature and natural environments create plenty of opportunities to be still and observe nature, which can also be a great source of epiphanic inspiration.

If you're uncomfortable with meditation, being quiet, or sitting still, start off slowly. Read a book while listening to nature sounds on a CD, or better yet, sit outside and read while you listen to the real thing. If you don't live near nature, find a park. If this is a problem, find a nature sounds station online that you can stream. Listen while you take a bath, lie down for a nap, or just before bed. Alternatively, try guided meditation. Check out the meditation video I've created at www.returnto-food.com/meditation. Slowly integrate one or more of these calming activities into your life.

Consider meditative walking in nature. Concentrate on your breathing. Other times, listen to inspiring information or talks or books on headphones while you're out walking. Both have benefits.

Be creative. Doodle, make crafts, write in your journal or in a notebook, even colour in a colouring book. Do what you initially feel comfortable with and observe what happens. As you bring more peace, quiet, and stillness into your life, you'll crave it more and more. You'll find your life is less stressful and fast-paced, too. Try to make this quiet time a part of your daily life.

CHAPTER EIGHT

THE HOLISTIC PATH

"When we know better, we do better."
Maya Angelou

FIND YOUR WHY

The *Return to Food* experience is different for everyone. I've found that people have the greatest success when they find a big enough *why*. Weight loss is rarely enough of a motivator, as there are deeper causes to be remedied than the amount of fat to lose. That *why* is different for everyone too and can be a combination of a few reasons. Ultimately, health, feeling good today and tomorrow, and living a long, good-quality life are some of the best reasons.

The important thing is to find a *why* that touches you emotionally and resonates with your deeper purpose in life. Losing weight to fit into a dress or suit for a wedding rarely works permanently as, once the wedding is over, the meaning is gone. Once you have a meaningful *why* in place and focus on it, your actions will be less arduous.

Once you've found your reason for change, you can move to the next step of preparing your kitchen for your new lifestyle. The recipes and resources in this book are here to guide you forward—and not just to use, but to have fun with. The kitchen can be the most delicious place of adventure and creation. Have fun with it.

KITCHEN AUDIT

A Kitchen Audit is a great tool in starting to set up a holistic kitchen. This is the process of removing the Lethal Recipe from your home and making room for nourishment. We go into this in the videos in the Return to Food online program, but below is the essence of it, if you are keen to get started.

Note: Before you start, a lot will come up for you around this exercise, for many reasons. If throwing out food was considered wasteful and a sin while you were growing up, then you may experience hesitation and even resistance. The important part to remember is that when you are throwing out the Lethal Recipe, you are not throwing out real food, just something that has the potential to make you sick.

When I was doing a kitchen audit in the home of a billionaire (who'd just spent over a $100,000 on a kitchen renovation), I went to throw out boxes of microwave popcorn full of GMO corn and chemicals. He resisted. He said he'd just use them up and then when they ran out, he'd buy organic popcorn. I told him he could afford to throw it out. In fact, because of the critical health issues he was facing, he couldn't afford not to.

If a billionaire has that reaction, you can imagine what comes up for people who are struggling to put food on their tables. Yet I've seen people who live for five years on what he spent on his kitchen renovations unwaveringly throw out the popcorn, because they knew the potential the Lethal Recipe had on their longevity and quality of life. What good is all our money if we don't live in a fit and vital body to enjoy it?

Every choice you make in the market, every bite you put in your mouth,
is a potential investment in your life.

AUDIT PROCEDURES

Start by placing what's in your cupboards and fridge into three categories on your kitchen table or wherever you have space:

Green	That which is easily obtained in nature; fresh vegetation.
Amber	That which is harder to find in nature: minimally processed meat, nuts, dairy; moderately processed food like whole grains and oils.
Red	That which cannot be obtained in nature, usually because the ingredients are highly processed or comprise a cocktail of the toxic five ingredients.

Lethal Recipe foods contain basic ingredients that have been processed in extreme conditions and/or have known toxic ingredients added. This category can include every food in the super-market—anything with refined sugar, oils, salt, and grains, and foods preserved or altered with chemicals for flavouring, colouring, and preserving.

Embrace the Green, Transition the Amber, and Avoid the Red

In almost every household I go to, the red category of foods is the largest area covering the table. It is an illuminating exercise for most people. Universally, as they move from decreasing and elimi-nating the red section from their household and their diet, and move toward the Amber with Green being the dominant section, symptoms of disease start to disappear. In the place of disease come vibrant energy, vitality, and well-being.

Try this for yourself at home: see what's in your cabinets and fridge. As you change your diet and lifestyle, aches, pains, and diseases will disappear, and vibrant, bountiful living will replace them.

Shopping

The best place to start shopping is your local farmers' market or any market that stocks primarily whole foods, has produce sections that sell organics, and has a good turnover.

Please support our organic and biodynamic farmers. The work they do is labour-intensive and honourable. I think of them as my kind heroes who are willing to work hard in a way that I am not. They take risks with growing their crops without agents that are harmful to the planet. You don't have to give them a handout. Just buy and promote their produce and thank them for their service to us and the planet.

Look online for what is local and for online delivery programs. CSAs (Community Shared Agriculture opportunities), Co-ops, local farmers, and Slow Food, a non-profit that offers alterna-tives to fast food, often list where you can get food locally. Even in the big-box supermarkets, you can ask for organic. Supermarkets will stock what people buy and eventually not stock what no one buys.

Growing your own food is a growing trend.

One of the best ways to return to food, to how we ate and sourced our food traditionally, is to grow your own garden, in your yard or in community plots. It's a growing trend (see what I did there?). There are also ways to cultivate food inside your home when the weather is inhospitable.

SETTING UP YOUR KITCHEN

The following is a basic outline of what I have in my kitchen.

DRY GOODS/THE PANTRY

- Pulses: lentils, peas, chickpeas, dried beans;
- Spices: my favourites are cumin, coriander, fennel seed, and Hontaka chili flakes.
- Cold-pressed coconut oil;
- Cold-pressed olive oil;
- Coconut palm sugar;
- Honey;
- Dried fruits: dates, prunes, raisins, sour cherries;
- Cacao;
- Mesquite;
- Lacuma;
- Maca;
- Whole vanilla bean powder;
- Sea salt;
- Pepper;
- Dried chili;
- Cumin;
- Coriander;
- Cinnamon;
- Ground ginger;
- Whole nutmeg seeds;
- Fennel seed;
- Fresh garlic;
- Fresh ginger.

THE FREEZER

- Seasonal berries;
- Fruit from summer;
- Stock cubes;
- Tomato sugo (sauce) made in late summer, early fall;
- Ice.

THE FRIDGE

- Nuts and seeds (raw): European almonds, hazelnuts, pumpkin seeds, sunflower seeds, unhulled sesame seeds;
- Vegetables;
- Fresh herbs, thyme, flat leaf parsley;
- Fruit that's in season;
- Sauerkraut—year round. I love it!
- Tamari—preferably wheat-free, organic;
- Miso paste;
- Apple cider vinegar.

EQUIPMENT

- Pots and pans—I use Saladmaster titanium cookware and love it.
- Knives—I have a mix of knives from over twenty-three years of professional cooking.
- ZuudleMaker—julienne vegetable slicer that makes the best raw zucchini noodles;
- Mason jars—love 'em for storing everything—the evolution from plastic;
- Microplane grater—my favourite is the flex stand-up one from The Pampered Chef[19];
- Vitamix—I love this blender!
- Kettle;
- Toaster;
- Chopping boards;

- Excalibur Dehydrator;
- The Travel Kitchen—see the video I created that I've shared with my private clients at www. returntofood.com/travelkitchen.

FROM LEARNING TO DOING

*Eating one apple is far more healthy and powerful than reading 1000 books on
how healthy an apple is.*

I had a client, Stella, who desperately wanted to lose weight and get healthy. Every day she'd scour the internet for the latest diet and trending nutritional information. She'd take courses with the latest expert who came into town, and buy new contraptions and concoctions that held out the promise of rapid weight loss and instant health. She had spent years researching, studying, and hiring experts to help her by the time she came to me. She had done everything except take action on the basic information that is encoded in our DNA—information we all know, but often resist applying—because that would make her let go of the behaviours that were comfortable and soothing, and keeping her stuck.

Learning is awesome, amazing, and … addictive. Education and preparation is a vital step in achieving anything. But at some point you have to do something, otherwise your preparation is in vain.

We can seek out new information to the point of distraction, and when it comes to nutrition and healthy eating, it can be another form of avoidance, just the way we can use food. Sadly, Stella is still overweight and suffering; "reading about apples" to avoid her resistance to just "eating the apple."

Arthur Schopenhauer said, "All truth passes through three stages. First it is ridiculed. Second it is violently opposed. Third it is accepted as being self-evident." I've experienced all these phases when presenting this concept over the years, since many of our present world's commercial interests that concern our lifestyle are its antithesis.

While I understand the value behind scientific validation, with all the wild claims out there and wacky products for sale that go along with them, I also have a belief that flies in the face of much of the scientific hierarchy related to health.

We are biological beings who are healthiest when we work synergistically with nature in its

143

natural state. The farther we deviate from and alter our natural environment, the sicker we and the planet become.

We have all that we need to heal the planet on this planet, and our task is not to reinvent nature, but to work with it in the most sustainable way, using our great wisdom to see and appreciate how to do this with little to NO effect on the environment for generations to come.

What is good for the body is good for the planet and what is good for the planet
is good for the body and every living species.

This feels like intuitive wisdom encoded in our DNA. I have seen the difference in people who harness nature and how vibrant and healthy they are by returning to food, as opposed to those buying pills and potions and gimmicks with claims of health.

You can wait for conclusive research to confirm that refined sugar is bad for you or you can give it up for thirty days and feel the difference that makes in your body and quality of life. Even a week will make a difference.

It's up to you. Wait for the years of research to show facts, stats, and data … or just try it yourself for thirty days and see the transformation begin. Observe how you feel physically, mentally, and emotionally.

If you've read this entire book and watched my recommended food documentaries, you've learned a better way to eat, think, and live. But knowing and doing are two different things. People often say they know better, so I ask why they are not eating better according to what information they have. Knowing is not just the result of taking in information and knowledge. It comes from experiencing, practising, falling down, and getting up. But mostly it comes from being present in your body, listening to the messages, and remembering what you want over the immediate gratification on the tongue and ensuing drug-like reactions.

One last bit of encouragement before you check out the recipes: to make the *Return to Food* transition with grace, remember to be kind and loving to yourself and others, from a place of strength. If someone makes this important change hard for you, understand it's about them, not you, and feel compassion. If you slip up and make poor food choices, I urge you to forgive yourself, recap your *why*, and get back on track to nourish your body, mind, heart, and soul. Living and eating the way we are meant to will give you a sense of connection with the universe and everything in it. Your holistic self will thank you, because you are worth the effort; your family and friends will thank you, because they love you. The planet will thank you, because you make it easier for it to give back.

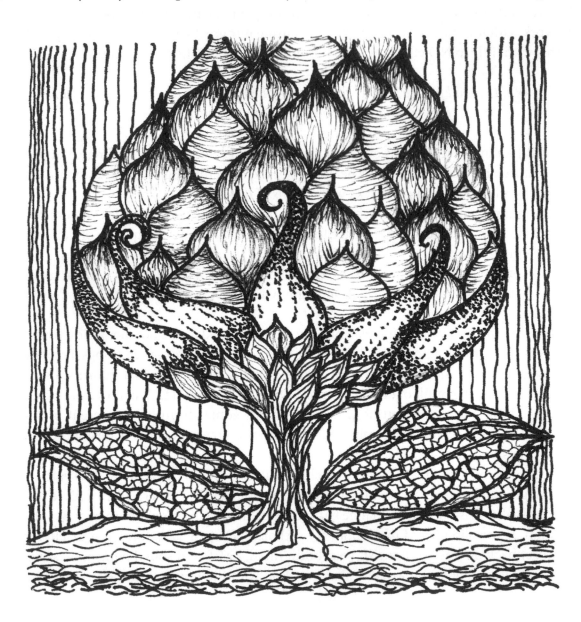

Recipes

Smoothies

WonderGreens Smoothie

Start with the fruit that is in season, particularly in summer. In the winter and autumn, you can always use apples and pears.

Ingredients
1 apple quartered and then halved (8 pieces), remove stem and core if you don't have a high-powered blender
1 kiwi fruit quartered
6 chopped leaves of kale or Black Tuscan cabbage (cavaleri nero) or 1 packed cup of fresh spinach or any dark greens like tatsoi
2 peeled cucumbers
Water to cover

Method
Blend in a high powered blender.
Drink right away but slowly.

Smoothie Variations
Avocado and 1 tbsp of raw cacao for a chocolate kick
Peaches, apricots, and nectarines in summer; make sure you pit them
Fresh or frozen berries—raspberries, blueberries, blackberries, huckleberries, and brambleberries, or a mixture of whatever is in season
Fresh pineapple
Frozen wheatgrass if you can get it at a health-food store
Sprouts for extra kick or a boost

Chocolove

Ingredients
1 cup raw almonds, soaked overnight (and peeled if you are energetic)
1 avocado
4 cups spring water
2 tsp maca powder
4 medjool dates soaked in 1 cup of water
2 tbsp raw cacao powder to taste
1 tsp vanilla powder
2 bananas, frozen,
1 tablespoon raw almond butter

Method
Place ingredients in the blender and blend until smooth.

Berry Bliss

Ingredients
All frozen
Blueberries, organic, wild
Mango
Banana
Spinach
Juice of 1 lime
Spring water

Method
Place ingredients in the blender and blend until smooth.

Veg In

Ingredients
Tomato, best in season
Spinach, herbs, basil, chilies
Kale, celery
Cucumber, in season
Zucchini
Spring water
optional, sea salt, Bragg's Liquid Aminos

Method
Place ingredients in the blender and blend until smooth.

Protein Passion

Ingredients
Avocado
Cinnamon, sprinkle
Vanilla powder
Handful dark green leaves
1 tbsp maple syrup or agave nectar
¼ cup hemp seeds raw
1 tbsp soaked chia seeds in ½ cup of spring water
Spring water

Method
Place ingredients in the blender and blend until smooth.

Salads

Glory Dressing

Do not be fooled by the simplicity of the ingredients—the magic is in choosing the best quality you can find, making sure it is organic and minimally processed.

Ingredients
4 tbsp apple cider vinegar, Bragg's brand is a universal favourite
4 tbsp cold-pressed organic olive oil (mix them up and vary the oils)
2 tbsp miso paste; make sure it is raw. Lighter-coloured miso pastes seem to work better—chickpea and white barley miso are my favourites

Method
Blend in high-powered blender. Drizzle and coat salad. Feel free to lick fingers ;-).

Teriyaki Dressing

Ingredients
1 tbsp organic tamari
1 tsp organic sesame oil
2 tbsp cold-pressed organic olive oil
2 tsp raw organic honey (coconut palm sugar for vegans)
2 tsp apple cider vinegar (optional for a tarter dressing with bite)
1 tsp of freshly grated ginger.
1 clove freshly grated garlic.

Method
Blend in high-powered blender. Drizzle and coat salad.

RAW CAESAR DRESSING

Ingredients
1 cup almonds, soaked and peeled
2 cloves fresh garlic
Juice of 1 large lemon
½ tsp salt
2 tbsp miso paste
½ tsp dulse
2 tbsp each of cold-pressed olive oil and water to create a mayonnaise consistency

Method
Blend to the consistency of mayonnaise, adding a little water at a time as you blend everything in a high-powered blender.
　Taste and add lemon to taste, adjusting seasoning.

BASIC VINAIGRETTE

Ingredients
¼ cup oil
¼ cup acid ingredient, like lemon juice or apple cider vinegar
1 garlic clove minced
1 tsp Dijon or seeded mustard or ground mustard seeds
Salt and pepper to taste

Method
Blend or shake to combine.

Variations Brainstorm
Tomato Vinaigrette
Seasonings
Making dressings from dips

Chickie Mix

Ingredients
250 gm sunflower seeds, toasted until golden
250 gm sesame seeds, toasted until golden
1 tbsp natural soy sauce
2 tsp sesame oil

Method
Either soak in marinade overnight and place in dehydrator until crunchy or lightly toast seeds on separate trays (sunflower seeds take longer).

If you are going to toast in the oven instead of marinating before cooking, after the seeds are toasted, evenly coat each tray of seeds with half each of the soy sauce and sesame oil (use a metal spatula).

Combine the two seeds. Cool. Place in an airtight container.

The Classic Big Bowl Salad

This is where it gets fun in the kitchen!
Below is simply a suggestion; open your mind to what is possible.

Ingredients
4 cups of mixed lettuces
6 kale leaves, thinly sliced
2 ripe tomatoes, diced, (in season)
1/6 cabbage, thinly sliced
2 baby carrots, washed and grated
1 beet, washed and grated
½ cup or generous handful of sunflower sprouts (they're my favourite now)
2 tbsp raw sunflower seeds
1 cup cooked rice blend

The Big Bowl Salad Variations

Be creative, think seasonal, always organic even if that means less is more; let go and connect to what you feel will nourish you in the moment.

Lettuces and greens—spinach, arugula/rocket, kales, cabbages, bok choy, chard, collard, dandelion greens.

Brightly coloured vegetables—beets, carrots, parsnip, celeriac, fennel, peppers, spring onions, leeks, cauliflower, broccoli, snow peas, beans ... there are hundreds to choose from. See what inspires you from the organic section of your market.

Good Fats—avocado, nuts and seeds, sunflower seeds, sesame seeds, pumpkin seeds, hemp hearts, coconut meat.

Fruits—tomatoes, cucumber, citrus fruits like lemon, lime, and grapefruit.

How to Make Zuudles

Zuudles are the fastest and best non-grain noodles, so simple and revolutionary when it comes to moving from refined grains to whole-food recipes.

Start with smaller, firmer zucchini about 6 inches in length and no more than 1.5 inches in width. You want them to be heavy for their size, and shiny and firm. I allow 1.5 per person or 2 for hungrier folk.

The massive zucchinis may look like a find, but as they grow larger, the flavour diminishes, and the texture is not good for perfect Zuudles.

Top and tail the zucchini. Translation: cut both ends off.

Don't peel the zucchini, as many of the precious nutrients are in the skin. I think it is the most delicious part with the best texture. It also adds a beautiful colour.

Take the zucchini lengthwise and firmly grate the whole length at a time to get long pasta-like strands. Work your way around the seeded centre of the zucchini and leave the centre to be chopped up and used however you like.

Epic Tree Hugger Salad with Zuudles

Ingredients
100 gm green beans
100 gm freshly shelled peas (snow, sugar snap, or English garden variety)
150 gm broccoli florets, sliced thinly
1 ripe avocado, sliced, optional
100 gm mixed lettuce leaves or spinach

Zuudles
4 small firm zucchini
Grate lengthwise on your ZuudleMaker or a Julienne Vegetable Slicer.

Teriyaki Dressing

Ingredients
1 tbsp organic tamari
1 tbsp unhulled sesame seeds
2 tbsp cold-pressed organic olive oil
2 tsp raw organic honey or coconut palm sugar
3 tsp of freshly grated ginger.
1 clove freshly grated or minced garlic.

Method
Blend, shake, or stir ingredients to create dressing.

Assembly
Gently toss all ingredients with the Teriyaki Dressing.

APPLE AND CARROT COOL SLAW

Ingredients
2 julienne-grated carrots
2 julienne-grated apples
1/3 cup raisins chopped
1/3 cup raw shelled walnuts or pecans, chopped
1 fresh lime, juice and zest of

Method
Squeeze lime juice over grated carrot, apple, and chopped raisins. Add the lime zest and walnuts. Gently toss ingredients together.

Don't be fooled by the low-key ingredients in this salad. It is super-simple, but deceptively delicious, great for breakfast, a fast snack, and even dessert.

Tips to Ensure the Best Cool Slaw
Of course, the ZuudleMaker Julienne Veg Slicer makes all the difference. Just as important and occasionally overlooked is the lime.

Make sure you have a fresh lime. In Canada, this can be a challenge! The best way to tell if you are going to have a great lime flavour is to scratch the lime and, if the zest gives off a beautiful lime scent, there's a big chance it will taste fabulous too. Always grate the apple last to reduce browning.

Brain Builder Salad

Ingredients

1 carrot, washed and grated
1 beetroot, washed and grated
1 yam, washed and grated
1 apple, washed and grated
1 ripe avocado, diced
Large handful of flat-leaf parsley, roughly chopped

Method

Lightly toss ingredients in a large salad bowl.
  Toss gently with dressing below.
  Sprinkle with sesame seeds for garnish.

Lemon Walnut Dressing

Ingredients

½ cup walnuts, soaked overnight in spring water or filtered water and then drained
juice from 2 lemons
2 tsp tamari or light soy sauce
½ tsp sea salt

Method

Blend on high in a blender until super smooth.

ZUUDLES WITH MISO GLORY DRESSING

Ingredients
4 small firm zucchini grated on a julienne strip slicer. See Zuudles instructions.
1 avocado sliced
1/3 cup raw, shelled walnuts (optional)

Method
Toss Zuudles with the Miso Glory Dressing.
    Arrange with sliced avocado and top with walnuts.

ZUUDLES WITH HEIRLOOM TOMATO DRESSING

Ingredients
2 whole raw cloves of garlic, minced or finely grated
4 ripe heirloom tomatoes (black Russians are a favourite or a variety of different-coloured tomatoes)
2 tbsp apple cider vinegar
1 tbsp hot water
½ tsp sea salt
2 tbsp cold-pressed olive oil
6 basil leaves, roughly chopped (optional)

Method
Dice the tomatoes, keeping all the juices. Add the remainder of the ingredients and mix well by hand, while still leaving chunks of tomato. You can use the back of a big spoon to squeeze the juice from the tomatoes.
    Add garlic, apple cider vinegar, hot water, sea salt, and cold-pressed olive oil.
    Lightly toss the Zuudles in the dressing until evenly coated. Serve with a smile!

Potato Salad

Ingredients
4 yams, whole, washed, and baked until tender
8 potatoes, whole, washed, and baked until tender
2 spring onions, finely sliced
4 eggs soft-boiled, optional or leave out for vegans
2 stalks of celery, diced

Method
Combine and dress with the Raw Caesar Dressing.

Lentil and Quinoa Salad

Ingredients
1 cup of lentils, soaked overnight and drained, simmered until just done
1 cup quinoa, cooked
½ cup chopped, soaked almonds
herbs
6 leaves of kale, sliced chiffonade (like julienne strips)
diced bell pepper
½ tsp cumin
salt and pepper to taste

Method
Gently combine with your favourite dressing.

Soups

Classic Pumpkin/Squash Soup

Ingredients
2 carrots, diced
2 sticks celery, diced
1 onion, diced
1 clove garlic, minced
1 tbsp coconut oil
1 kg of butternut pumpkin/squash, peeled and diced
3 sprigs of thyme
Salt and pepper to taste

Method
Sauté mirepoix (chopped celery, onions, and carrots) in coconut oil until softened. Add garlic for an additional few minutes.

Add pumpkin, thyme, salt, and pepper. Cover with water. Gently simmer until pumpkin softens to the point of breaking down. Blend half the soup and add back in.

Variations can include the addition of spices and ginger.

Ginger Miso and Tahini Broth (GMT Broth)

Ingredients
4 tbsp miso paste
2 tbsp unhulled tahini
3 square inches of grated ginger

Method
Mix to a paste.

Lightly simmer vegetables in just enough water to cover. Remove from heat once vegetables are wilted.

Take 4 tbsp of water out and mix into miso paste. Pour mixture back into the vegetables in the water.

Taste and adjust.

Additions and Variations for GMT Broth
Add 1 tsp of coconut palm sugar
Add 1 tbsp of juice from tamarind paste
Add a pinch of Hontaka chili pepper
Vegetables that work best—Asian greens like wombok, bok choy and gai lan, broccoli, savoy cabbage, mushrooms
Rice and quinoa are also good fillers for hungry eaters.

CELERIAC LEEK AND LENTIL SOUP

Ingredients
2 small leeks, washed and sliced
1 tbsp organic butter
1 tbsp cold-pressed olive oil
1 celeriac, peeled and diced
1 potato, washed and diced
1 cup green lentils
Water to cover
1 tsp sea salt
1 tbsp raw miso paste (it is worth searching for chickpea miso, and you can also use it to make your own salad dressings)
Fresh cracked pepper
Handful of spinach, optional

Method
Gently sauté leeks in butter and olive oil. Add celeriac, lentils, and potato. Cover with water and simmer until potato and lentils are tender. Season with sea salt and pepper.

Add rocket or spinach once off the heat (fresh green leaves)

Pulse blend to finish with a stick blender or place one third of the soup in a blender or food processor until smooth in consistency and add back to the soup.

Variations
Broccoli—replace cauliflower with broccoli; use the whole head and peeled stem
Carrot—grate garden-fresh, baby carrots in place of the cauliflower
Beet—grate whole, washed beets in place of cauliflower
Sweet potato—replace potatoes with sweet potato or yams
Butternut squash or pumpkin—replace cauliflower with butternut squash/pumpkin
Cauliflower—use a whole head and break into florets
Garden greens—prepare the soup above and once off the heat add in garden greens—podded peas, fava beans, green beans, asparagus and leafy greens—for a delicious, garden delight.

Sweet Potato, Black Kale, Black Bean Soup

Ingredients
Spring or filtered water to cover ingredients
2 small carrots, diced
1 small onion, diced
1 stick of celery, diced
1 half leek, washed and sliced
1 clove of garlic, minced
1 tbsp cold-pressed coconut oil
1 tsp ground fennel
1 tsp ground cumin
1 tsp ground coriander
¼ tsp ground pepper
1 medium potato, diced
1 medium sweet potato, diced
1 cup cooked black beans
3 sprigs of thyme
1 tsp natural salt
4 leaves of black Tuscan kale, thinly sliced (also called Italian kale or dinosaur kale)

Method
In at least a 3-litre saucepan, sauté carrots, onion, celery, leek, and garlic in coconut oil for 5 minutes, on a low heat. Add spices and sauté for 3 minutes.

Add potato, sweet potato, black beans, thyme, and salt. Cover in water about 1 cm over the top of ingredients.

Simmer over a low temperature until the potatoes are tender and easily broken. When soup is thick and potatoes are falling apart, remove from heat and stir in chopped kale. Serve and enjoy.

Grains and Grain-Like Things

Apple Porridge

Ingredients
See measurements in method
Rolled oats
Apples of your choice
Cinnamon
Fresh shelled nuts, sultanas, fresh almond milk (optional)

Method
Allow 1/3 cup of organic rolled oats per person for breakfast, ½ cup for big eaters.

Soak in double the amount of water overnight—so for 1/3 cup of oats, use 2/3 cups of water; a pinch of sea salt and a squeeze of lemon will help make the nutrients more bioavailable.

Dice 1 apple per person. Place into a pot with a lid and sprinkle with cinnamon. Steam with lid on until apple is tender; this varies depending on the variety. When apples are done, remove and add oats to the pot and cook until thick and congealed, about 4 minutes; 6 minutes if there is a large volume.

Top with fresh shelled nuts, sultanas, and fresh almond milk.

Swiss Brown Mushroom Risotto

Ingredients
1 red onion
1 clove garlic
2 tbsp organic first cold-pressed extra virgin olive oil
2 cups water
4 sprigs of thyme
1 cup biodynamic brown rice
400 gm of the most flavourful mushrooms you can find, sliced thinly
2 large handfuls of spinach
sea salt and pepper to taste

Method
Sauté onion in olive oil until tender. Add mushrooms and garlic, and sauté until mushrooms collapse and start to release juices.

Add rice and continue to sauté for 2 minutes. Add thyme and water to cover; simmer until rice is al dente, about 45 minutes. Remove from heat and stir in spinach until wilted. Season to taste.

Optional
Add miso for a cheesy flavour.
Garnish with herbs like parsley, green onion, or chives.

Quinoa, Kale, and Parsley Salad

Ingredients
Cooked quinoa
Kale, chopped and massaged
Italian flat-leaf parsley, roughly chopped
Leek, finely sliced
Cucumber, diced
Bell pepper, diced
Grated carrot
Lemon juice
Olive oil
Salt and pepper

Method
Gently combine all ingredients with your favourite dressing.

Buckwheat Granola

Method and Ingredients
1 cup buckwheat, water to soak overnight. Drain buckwheat in the morning and rinse well. Soak again for at least 2 hours with ¼ tsp cinnamon, freshly grated nutmeg to taste, ¼ tsp orange zest, and water to soak.

Drain again thoroughly and marinate in ¼ cup agave nectar, ¼ tsp cinnamon, ¼ tsp vanilla bean powder, 2 dates pitted and finely chopped, 2 tsp maca powder, ¼ tsp sea salt.

Add 1 cup of mixed nuts and seeds that are soaked overnight and drained to the drained buckwheat seeds with chopped dried fruit in the agave mixture.

Coat evenly. Lay the mixture on dehydrator trays and dehydrate for 12 hours or until crunchy, or bake slowly at 200° C until golden.

Serve with almond milk or tossed through grated apple and carrot.

Stock Concentrate (Adapted From a Thermomix Recipe)

Ingredients
200 gm celery, roughly chopped
2 carrots, roughly chopped
1 onion, peeled and quartered
1 tomato, quartered
1 small zucchini, tightly chopped
2 cloves garlic, peeled
4 sprigs of thyme leaves
2 bay leaves fresh, chop a few leaves of basil, rosemary, and sage
1 bunch of Italian flat-leaf parsley, roughly chopped
150 gm sea salt
1 tbsp cold-pressed coconut oil

Method
Purée ingredients in high-speed blender, Vitamix, or Thermomix until smooth.

Place spoonfuls into ice cube trays and freeze. Remove from trays when frozen and store in the freezer in an airtight container.

Pull out a cube or two to season soups or anywhere you would normally use a stock seasoning.

Pulses

Lentil Stew

Ingredients
2 sticks celery, diced
2 carrots, diced
1 large onion, diced
1 tbsp coconut oil
3 sprigs thyme
300 ml cooked tomatoes
1 cup lentils, soaked
2 cups finely sliced cabbage
4 small potatoes diced
water to cover
salt and pepper to taste
2 tsp apple cider vinegar, optional

Method
Sauté celery, carrots, and onion in coconut oil until tender. Add the remaining ingredients, except for vinegar, and simmer until potatoes are tender. Finish with vinegar and seasoning to taste.

Caramelized Onion and Chickpea Soup

Ingredients
4 onions, thinly sliced
1 tbsp olive oil
1 tbsp butter
1 cup of chickpeas, soaked and drained
3 sprigs rosemary
Sea salt and pepper to taste

Method
Sauté onions in oil and butter until tender and caramelized.
   Add chickpeas and rosemary.
   Cover with water to about 4 cm above chickpeas.
   Simmer for about 1.5 hours.
   Season with salt and pepper to taste.

DHAL BABY

Ingredients
2 cups red lentils, soaked
1 inch knob of ginger, grated
2 cloves of garlic, minced
2 cm fresh turmeric, grated
1 large onion diced
2 tsp cumin, ground
generous pinch of dried chili
2 tsp mustard seeds
1 tsp sea salt
2 tbsp coconut oil
juice of half a lemon
fresh coriander/cilantro

Method
Sauté onion until tender. Add ginger, garlic, turmeric, cumin, mustard seeds, chili, and sauté for another 2 minutes. Add lentils and cover with water and simmer for about 30 minutes, stirring regularly.

Finish by seasoning with salt, a squeeze of lemon, and freshly chopped coriander leaves.

Stews & Casseroles

Cauliflower, Leek & Potato Casserole

Ingredients

2 leeks, washed and sliced
2 tbsp olive oil, cold-pressed
4 potatoes, large dice
½ cauliflower, divided into florets
4 sprigs of thyme
4 kale leaves, sliced
2 tsp salt and fresh cracked pepper
Water to cover
A handful of flat-leaf parsley, roughly chopped

Method

Sauté leeks in olive oil under tender. Add the rest of ingredients except parsley and kale. Cook until tender over a low heat.

Once tender, garnish with chopped parsley.

Optional

Once off the heat, add 4 kale leaves, sliced; stir through as you add the parsley.

Split Pea and Root Stew

Ingredients
1 onion, diced
2 carrots, diced
2 yams/sweet potatoes
1 swede/turnip, peeled and diced
1 parsnip, diced
1 cup split peas, soaked overnight
2 bay leaves
½ tsp white pepper
1 cup stewed tomatoes
1 cup cooked chickpeas
1 tsp salt

Method
Place all ingredients in a casserole dish with just enough water to cover. Simmer on low until vegetables are very tender. Remove bay leaves and serve.

Smokey Eggplant, Celeriac, and Mushroom Casserole

Ingredients
2 onions, diced and caramelized
300 gm crimini mushrooms, sliced in half
1 eggplant, smoked
1 celeriac, peeled, diced
½ tsp ground fennel seed
3 tbsp olive oil, cold-pressed
2 cloves garlic, minced
1 cup du puy lentils
2 zucchini, grated

Method
Sauté onion, mushroom, celeriac, fennel seed, and garlic in olive oil for 5 minutes. Add zucchini and lentils, cover with water and simmer on low. When the celeriac and lentils are tender, gently add the smoked eggplant at the end.

Smokey Eggplant

Method and Ingredients
1 eggplant charred over a flame until tender inside. Split in half and scoop out tender flesh. Add minced clove of garlic, olive oil, sea salt, pepper, and a squeeze of lemon. Gently chop and fold in the above ingredients to create a smoky topping to the soup.

Gluten-Free Baking and Holistic Sweets

Sweet Potato (Yam) Date Muffins (12 Units)

This recipe was made by my dear friend Viv who came and taught at the Return to Food Academy.

Ingredients
1¾ cups organic quinoa flour
1 tsp baking powder
1 tsp baking soda
¼ tsp seat salt
¼ to ½ tsp ground nutmeg
1 tsp cinnamon
1/3 cup organic extra virgin coconut oil
1/3 cup organic coconut sugar
2 tbsp organic agave nectar
2 large eggs
2 cups mashed, cooked sweet potato (yams)
¾ cup chopped pitted dates

Method
Preheat the oven to 375°F. Lightly grease a 12-cup muffin pan or line with parchment liners.

In a large bowl, whisk together the quinoa flour, baking powder, soda, salt, nutmeg, and cinnamon. In a medium bowl, cream the coconut oil, coconut sugar, and maple syrup. Beat in the eggs, one at a time. Whisk in the sweet potato. Add this to the flour mixture and stir just until blended. Add the dates; mix until well distributed. Scoop the batter evenly among the muffin cups.

Bake for 18 to 20 minutes or until a toothpick inserted into the centre of a muffin comes out clean. Cool in the pan for about 5 minutes, then remove.

Jiivala's Hot Choc VGF Brownies

Jiivala Holistic Culinary Academy was the precursor to the Return to Food Academy. These brownies are wonderful ways to segue off dairy and ice creams that have processed sugar. You will need a high-powered blender; a food processor will work in a pinch, but the texture will not be as creamy.

Ingredients
1 cup hot water
½ tsp baking soda
6 dates, pitted
½ cup coconut palm sugar
½ cup coconut oil
1 tsp vanilla bean powder
1½ cup ground almonds*
¾ cup cocoa powder
½ cup chopped walnuts
¼ cup chopped dark chocolate or choc chips

Method
Add baking soda to hot water and pour over dates. Cool date mix/paste and blend with coconut palm sugar, coconut oil, vanilla bean powder.

  Sift cocoa with ground almonds. Fold through cocoa and almonds mix with date paste. Fold in nuts and chocolate.

  Pour into mini muffin top tins. Bake for 10 minutes or until just cooked through.

Mango Banana Nice Cream

Ingredients
½ cup frozen banana chunks
½ cup frozen mango chunks
Fresh squeezed juice from 1 blood orange or 1 lime

Method
Take chunks of frozen fruit and blend them in a high powered blender until smooth and creamy. To help the blending process you can combine fresh squeezed juice to also add flavour.

Peach, Grape, and Passion Fruit Sorbet

Ingredients
1 cup frozen peach chunks
1 cup frozen grapes
4 tbsp of passion fruit juice

Method
Blend until soft, serve sorbet texture.

MACAROONIES

Ingredients
2 cup shredded, raw, unsweetened coconut
½ cup ground raw almonds (or almond flour)
½ agave syrup or coconut palm sugar for caramel flavour
2 tbsp coconut oil
1 tsp vanilla powder
1/8 tsp sea salt

Method
Mix all ingredients together in a bowl, till dough comes together to form ball shapes easily.
Scoop in tablespoons onto a lined dehydrator tray for 7 hours or overnight at 110° C, or bake on 250° C for one hour or 325° C for 15 minutes.

Variations
Chocolate: add cacao to taste
Mint: a few drops of mint oil to taste
Spirulina for green colouring
ChocoMint: Divide the batch in half and make one mint and one chocolate and then press the mint on top of the chocolate layer.
Variation on the ChocoMint: Dip mint macaroons in melted chocolate.
Raspberry: Add 1 tbsp or dried raspberry powder
Lime: Juice and zest from 1 lime. Sprinkle of spirulina for the green colour

JIIVALA APPLE MUFFINS

Ingredients

1 cup Anita's sprouted spelt flour
1 tsp baking powder (aluminum free)
1 tsp cinnamon
1 grated apple
2 eggs
1 tsp vanilla
70 gm melted organic salted butter
1 cup of almond milk (you can use any milk)
½ cup honey

Method

Sift together dry ingredients. Whisk together rest of ingredients. In each muffin tin, place a dob of butter in the bottom of the pan; sprinkle with coconut palm sugar.

Add apple slices plus 7 cups of love stirred into each step.

Fold wet into dry ingredients and spoon over apples in tins and bake until muffin centres are cooked through, about 15 minutes for muffin tops, and 25-30 for normal sized muffins.

Dips and Sauces

Pad Thai Sauce

Ingredients

4 tbsp Miso
3 inches ginger, grated on microplane grater
1 tsp dulse flakes
2 tbsp coconut sugar
1 cup tahini
¼ tsp chili

Method

Whisk or blend until smooth. Add water to create desired sauce consistency.

Sweet n Spicy Tomato Sauce

Ingredients

500 ml stewed tomatoes or tomato sugo
3 dates soaked in 1/3 cup of water
1/3 cup sun-dried tomatoes (soaked with dates overnight)
¼ cup cold-pressed oil
¼ tsp Hontaka chili flakes
1 tsp ruby salt
1 tbsp apple cider vinegar

Method

Blend in Vitamix until smooth.

Basic Hummus

Ingredients
2 cups chickpeas, soaked and cooked until tender
2 cloves of garlic juice of 1 large lemon
3 tbsp tahini
1.5 tsp salt
2 tbsp cold-pressed olive oil

Method
Blend in high-powered blender until smooth and creamy.

Variations
Roasted garlic
Roasted red pepper, skinned
1 tbsp miso paste
Soaked chipotle pepper
Ground coriander and cumin

Rosemary, Roasted Garlic, and White Bean Dip

Ingredients
1 head of garlic, sliced in half and roasted until soft and golden (this can take up to an hour and longer for elephant garlic). Slice the bulb in half and place flat side down on an oiled baking tray)
2 cups of presoaked white beans cooked until tender with a sprig of rosemary
1 onion, sliced and sautéed.
1 tbsp cold-pressed olive oil
Salt to taste
Fresh cracked pepper

Method
Purée beans with roasted garlic that has been squeezed out of its skin. Finish with a drizzle of cold-pressed oil and chopped flat-leaf parsley.

Raw and Dehydrated

Spicy Avocado Soup

Ingredients
2 avocados, ripe
¾ of a medium cucumber
1 stalk celery, finely diced
Juice of 1 lime
Small handful of fresh coriander (cilantro)
2 tsp ground cumin
1 tsp ground coriander seeds
½ tsp sea salt
¼ tsp chili flakes
1 tsp tamari
1 cup water (if wanting warm soup use hot water)

Method
Blend all ingredients in a high-speed blender until smooth. Transfer to a serving bowl and finish with finely chopped green onions.

Veggie Chips

Ingredients
Thinly sliced vegetables
Kale
Zucchini
Sweet potato/yam
Beetroot
Carrot
Lemon juice
Sea salt
Olive oil
Crushed pepper or ground spices to taste

Method
Coat vegetables with salt, olive oil, and lemon juice. Make sure it is evenly but sparingly coated.
   Dehydrate until crisp. Different vegetables take different times; kale takes about 8 hours and beet chips can take up to 14 hours.

Apple Chips

Ingredients
Apples
Cinnamon
Lemon juice

Method
Coat apple slices in lemon juice and cinnamon to taste. Dehydrate overnight, about 8–12 hours, until crispy.

Key Lime Truffles from Joy McCarthy
(www.joyoushealth.com)

One of my students, Semhar, introduced me to this recipe and I'm an absolute convert.

Ingredients
1 ripe avocado
Juice and zest of 1 lime
½ cup organic coconut oil
¼ cup honey
½ cup shredded coconut (look for organic and unsulfured)

Method
Peel and remove the seed of the avocado. Place into food processor. Squeeze the juice of the lime on top of the avocado and add the lime zest. Melt the coconut oil over medium heat, then add to the food processor. Add the honey and blend until completely smooth.

Transfer to a bowl and place in freezer for one hour or until it's solid enough to form into balls. Place the shredded coconut into a bowl. Spoon out the avocado mixture and form into balls.

(Note: The balls won't be perfectly round, but once you roll in the coconut shreds they'll form better.)

Place rolled balls back into the freezer for a couple of hours.

Apple Crumble

Ingredients of Crumble Topping
1 cup raw pecans
½ cup fresh shelled walnuts
4 pitted fresh dates
1 tsp vanilla bean powder
½ tbsp cold-pressed coconut oil

Method
In a food processor, combine all ingredients until they become crumbly.

Ingredients of Filling
6 medium-sized McIntosh or heirloom variety, soft-fleshed apples (2 for pureeing / 4 sliced)
Apple Sauce
2 pitted fresh dates
¼ cup raisins
1 tsp cinnamon
2 tsp raw honey or agave nectar
1 tbsp fresh squeezed lemon juice
½ tsp vanilla extract
¼ tsp fresh grated nutmeg
½ tsp vanilla bean powder

Method
Reserve 4 apples for the bulk filling. Purée 1 peeled apple with the rest of the ingredients until smooth. Slice the 4 apples or dice as preferred. Marinate in the apple sauce.

Top apples in crumble mixture.

ALMOND MILK

Ingredients
1 cup almonds raw
2 pitted dates
¼ tsp vanilla bean powder or half a vanilla bean

Method

Soak almonds in plenty of filtered or spring water overnight. If you have the energy, peel the almonds as the milk will be creamier and there will be fewer antinutrients from the skins. In nature, when you peel a fresh almond it comes out of its shell without the skin. The skin reattaches to the almonds so that it can be stored and will not sprout until it's reactivated with moisture.

Drain water in the morning and add 4 cups of spring or filtered water, fresh dates, and ½ vanilla bean, finely chopped.

Allow to sit for at least 2 hours to allow the date to break up and the vanilla bean to soften.

Blend in a blender at highest speed until the mix is very smooth. Serve with chia pudding as is or if you prefer a true milk texture, strain the liquid from the pulp through a nut milk bag or strain through cheesecloth over a mesh strainer.

Variations
Alcash Milk—Add cashews for a creamier nut milk
Cinnamon Milk—Add a tsp of cinnamon
Chocolove—Add 1 tbsp of raw cacao
Omega Boost—½ cup hemp seeds for higher protein content
Eggless Nog—½ tsp cinnamon, ¼ ground cloves, ½ tsp ground nutmeg
Orange Vanilla—1 tsp of orange zest and 1 tsp vanilla powder
Replace the dates with 1 tbsp of raw honey and 1 tsp of vanilla powder.

Fermenting

Sauerkraut

This recipe was adapted from a former student and now delightful friend, Nikoo, who came to teach at the academy. Sauerkraut and other fermented vegetables have many amazing health benefits, are easy and affordable to make, and are a sustainable way of preserving local, fresh vegetables.

Ingredients
1 head of cabbage, red or green
1-2 tbsp sea salt
2 tsp dill seed
6 cloves of garlic

Tools
1 litre wide-mouth Mason jar
Large bowl to hold vegetables for pounding

Method
Slice the cabbage into thin strips. Place in a large bowl. Add 1 tbsp of salt to the cabbage.

Massage, grind, knead, and pound the cabbage thoroughly with your hands and fists, or a heavy pestle. As the cabbage gets worked, the salt will draw water out of it. This may take some time, so be patient and have fun with it.

Taste a piece of cabbage. You want it to be salty, resembling salty ocean water. If it does not taste salty enough, add another half-tbsp of salt and continue massaging. Massage until the cabbage is submerged in its own juices.

Place the massaged cabbage and all the juice into the Mason jar. With your fist or clean utensil, press down the cabbage until it is submerged under the juice. If not fully submerged, add a bit of spring water.

Rub a lemon on the surface of the cabbage and around the lip of the jar. This prevents surface mould from forming. Place the lid on the jar. It does not have to be airtight. If the lid is airtight, leave at least 3 inches of space at the top of the jar (because fermentation produces gases).

Place the jar in a dark, warm place. The vegetables will start to ferment within days, but will get stronger and more potent (with beneficial micro-organisms, vitamins, and flavour) with time.

Let it sit for at least 1 week, and up to 4 weeks. You can open the lid and taste a bit of sauerkraut with a clean utensil to see if it has developed a pleasant tart and tangy flavour. Once the sauerkraut has reached a taste that you enjoy, or after 1 to 4 weeks, place it in the refrigerator. It can now be scooped out for use at will.

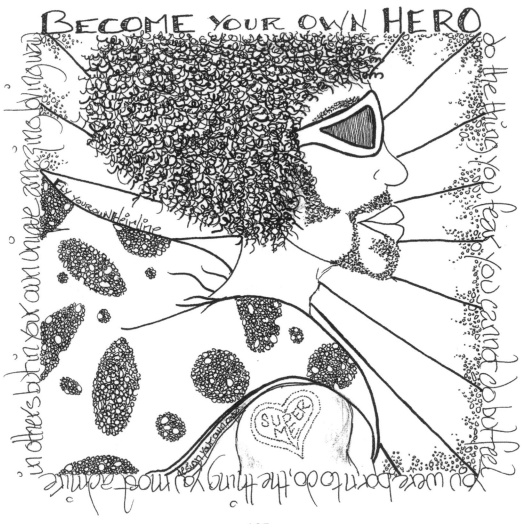

THE HOLISTIC HERO'S JOURNEY

During several decades of witnessing thousands of people on their journey to health, I noticed a pattern of behaviours, which I came to realize mirrors author Joseph Campbell's hero's journey. This pattern comprises what I call the eleven stages of the Holistic Hero's Journey. When you can see the path, like looking at a map, you can see where you've been, where you are, and where you're heading. This can bring you comfort on a challenging journey. But understanding where you are can actually fast-track your progress through awareness.

BLISSFULLY OR PAINFULLY UNAWARE

At this stage, you have no idea of how food plays a part in how you are feeling and your energy levels. You may be eating the Lethal Recipe and, due to great genetics or a positive mental and emotional frame of mind, you are not experiencing symptoms of disease. Alternatively, you may be experiencing chronic pain due to disease and be painfully unaware that how you are eating is a major contributor to your state of health.

INFORMATION TO KNOWLEDGE

A seed has been planted and you are starting to gather information and knowledge, alerting you to your ignorance and enlightening you as to how you may potentially reverse your symptoms of lethargy, excess weight, or disease. You acknowledge a separation from nature that has led to your pain and/or disease state, and you start to feel a calling to change.

RESISTANCE

You feel a calling to change, but may feel broken and not up to it, and you refuse the call. You get a sense of everything involved in recognizing that the world as you know it is not quite right. Think of the character Neo in The Matrix . This is the stage at which you realize all that is involved in the process of switching from your present toxic state to that of a "Holistic Hero," and you resist, usually due to being overwhelmed and fearful of the death of a life you've become accustomed to, even if it is making you sick and killing you.

Becoming Aware

In the stage of awareness, you've started to make some changes that cause shifts in your body and how you are feeling. This is where mentors and teachers appear to guide you in the form of books, films, videos, and people who've been on the path.

Awakening

This is the "religious" stage, when you exhibit the zeal of the newly converted. Your transformation has been an "I've seen the light" experience. You have more energy, your pain is gone or greatly diminished, your disease symptoms have reversed, your blood sugar and blood pressure are normal. There is no going back and you are committed to change.

You tend to be black and white about choices. There is a danger of being judgmental, of exerting a bit of superiority over others now that you have seen the light. You want to share this with the world, as it seems all the others around you are deluded and drinking the Kool-Aid (literally and figuratively!).

You are most likely given to fads in this stage, and the cleaner and more extreme, the better. You are on the bandwagon and most likely suffering from information addiction. You find it hard not to spread the word, and realize that almost every conversation can be turned into one about your new way of eating. It is also not surprisingly the most likely stage to repel people, so be mindful and gentle with them; think long-term, and think of the expression, "I prefer to be kind versus right." People will be more inspired by how you look and feel than by what you tell them, especially if you tell them from a position of "nutritional moral superiority."

SHIFTING

In this stage, there is an acceptance fuelled by the motion that was generated by the emotion and ensuing energy of the Awakening Stage. You start to experiment with what works for you. There are ever-present temptations and dangers, and you are no longer so emotional in your approach. You move toward mental intellectualizing, which can make things feel like hard work. Logic steps in, faddish behaviours start to lose their shine, and you start the process of figuring out what really works for you.

TURNING

This is the stage at which you start the internal evolution to mirror the external. You start the upward spiral of emotions that vibrate at a higher level, and as a result you frequently make choices that give you more energy. It is not easy, but not too difficult, and you know you can never truly go back to the Lethal Recipe. Yet this is the stage of potentially falling back to the old patterns and behaviours, or at least questioning the call to return to food, too. But your body is now accustomed to what it is like to eat nourishing foods, and so the contrast is very much in your awareness.

HABITUATING

You are no longer propelled by zeal and some routines can become boring, but you are committed. You are coming out of an initiation of sorts and there is a clear death of the old way of being. You may mourn for old foods and rituals that brought you comfort, and struggle to form new ones that serve you. You also struggle with the thoughts and ensuing emotions that you inevitably feel when you are no longer using the Lethal Recipe to numb, push down, or bliss out. It might be a struggle to move through and develop truly empowering tools to evolve past old patterns and thoughts that are not serving you.

MAINTAINING

You've finally fully accepted your new path. You have taken the torch and are running with it. You've fully accepted the consequences and the transformation into a new life. Temptations come, but you are much more able to resist them and are more forgiving toward yourself when you do revert to former behaviours.

LIVING

This is the stage of clear, conscious choice. You've worked through the angst and done the time and the work to get to a place of contentment. You are eating in a way that is right for your body, your way of being, and your values. It is much easier to resist the things that don't serve you, and making those better choices is just a matter of you saying and believing, "This is how I do life." You feel as though you've atoned for the transgressions against your body and the environment and have no need to make others feel inferior to you because of their choices. At this stage, you will inspire people to enquire about your change.

BEING

This is the stage of total acceptance of self and true peace around your choices. Your way of being is so nonjudgmental and your vibration is so elevated that others just "want" to eat and live better because of how good they feel around you, without your saying a word. Food can still bring you pleasure, but there is no obsession or dependency on food for pleasure. You are able to find pleasure in the thoughts you choose and the emotions and empowerment that this brings.

This is where you have a deeper insight into the journey from the place where you were ignorant. That journey took you into a special world previously unknown to you (and many people who orbit around you). You gained information, insights, experience, and wisdom that elevated your physical, mental, emotional, and spiritual being. You've returned from this journey and realized that you were never actually broken, just unaware. You marvel at how amazing you were in each stage and at the relevance of each stage along the way in relation to next. You revel in the return to the known world where you are now entrusted to bring this amazing knowledge to others. As you advance through this stage, you become aware of another part of your life where you experience a limited awareness, and your next journey begins.

The Being Stage isn't about perfection, but rather about a state of peace with your journey and the measure of your health, which is a reflection of eating in a more nourishing, energizing, and protective way for your body and the planet .

People transcend in different ways, at different times, and on different levels. The eleven stages are a guide only, so be aware of the folly of comparison; no two journeys are exactly alike. We all have different challenges and life experiences that bring us to each phase and stage in our own way and timing.

It is not uncommon to span different stages as we spiral up to a higher vibrational frequency. You may need to spend much more time in one phase than in another as you transition fully into it. Some people transcend all the phases quickly, either because their situation is life-threatening or they're in extreme pain or simply through a miracle. No matter where you are, please be kind to yourself and others.

On your entire journey, self-awareness is a great tool for advancing with greater ease and grace. Also, find the places where you can experience the most elevated forms of joy, where you can move into a compassionate place of love for yourself and then others. That is the fastest, most graceful way to return to food with love for your body and the planet.

Afterword

"God grant me the serenity
to accept the things I cannot change;
courage to change the things I can;
and wisdom to know the difference."
Reinhold Niebuhr

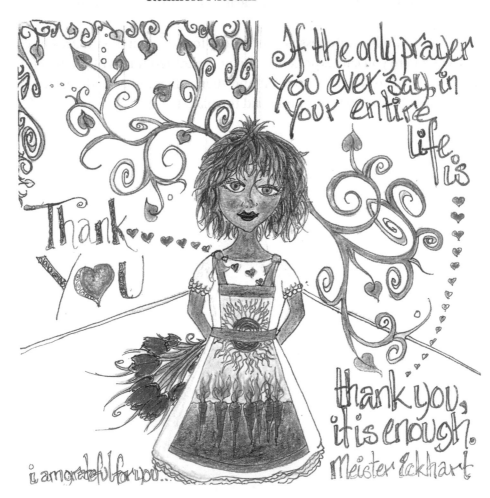

Gratitude is the final piece of the *Return to Food* anti-diet. I simply cannot find adequate words to express how it has transformed every area of my life. It continues to be the practice that drives every good thing in my life forward. I remember a time when people said a prayer or gave thanks for what they were about to eat. A time when we would say a blessing, conscious of what the earth provided, what sacrifices occurred so that we may eat; for farmers who tended the soil, animals that were sacrificed, hands that tended the earth, watered plants, harvested and gathered as a loving act of service, sometimes through blood, sweat and tears.

I'm deeply grateful for thousands of people who've crossed my path with conversations, lessons, and experiences that have enriched and refined my life and ultimately shaped and influenced how I see the world and food.

I'm grateful for every mouthful of food that has ever crossed my lips, close and far from nature; it has all been a classroom for me, with powerful lessons that brought tears, pain, joy, and delight to my palate, body, and soul. I'm grateful for the loving connections at the table, both sober and tipsy. For every nutrient that has nourished and protected my body. Conversations that took me beyond my narrow world view, touched my heart, and opened my eyes. For every pound of fat, gained and lost. My incredibly amazing body that always moves toward healing. For where I live, the path I've chosen, and how it gives me access to incredibly delicious produce. For farmers who risk growing without pesticides and who build the soil instead of poison it, who go out in inhospitable weather and travel to the markets to sell me what they've produced with integrity and pride. For my students and teachers who are both my teachers and students; I am always amazed how every moment in life is an opportunity to learn.

For every meal that has created connection, conversation, and community. For the silence between bites, meals shared and in solitude. For the practice of being present for what I am eating (I'm still learning). For the sensuous nature of food that weaves its magic on what appears to be many dimensions, textures, flavours, colours, and aromas. For the nourishment that keeps me grounded and the ingredients that grant me bliss.

For the most amazing, loving, wise, funny, and kind students, teachers, and mentors who push me to be more authentic, real, honest, and to love without fear. For everyone who reads these words and passes on what they learned through sharing a thought, a snack, a meal, or conversation that just may save or enrich a life.

In service and depth of gratitude,
Sherry Strong

Resources

Books

Over the years I've bought hundreds of books, so a list at the end of this book seems impossible to curate. Here are a few that stick in my mind as must-haves:

- Kris Carr, *Crazy Sexy Kitchen*, Hay House, 2012
- Kris Carr, *Crazy Sexy Cancer Survivor*, Globe Pequot Press, 2008
- Dr. Gabriel Cousens, *Conscious Eating*, North Atlantic Books, 2000
- Charles Eisenstein, *The More Beautiful World Our Hearts Know is Possible*, North Atlantic books, 2013
- Charles Eisenstein, *The Yoga of Eating*, Newtrends Publishing, 2003
- Udo Erasmus, *Fats that Heal, Fats that Kill*, Alive Books, 1993
- Mariel Hemingway, *Finding My Balance*, Simon & Schuster, 2004
- Mariel Hemingway and Bobbie Williams, *Running with Nature*, Changing Lives Press, 2013
- Jena LaFlamme, *Pleasurable Weight Loss*, Sounds True, 2015
- Yotam Ottolenghi, *Plenty*, Chronicle Books, 2011
- Yotam Ottolenghi, *Plenty More*, Ten Speed Press, 2014
- Geneen Roth, *Women, Food and God*, Scribner, 2010
- Julia Rothman, *Farm Anatomy*, Storey Publishing, 2011
- Marianne Williamson, *Return to Love*, HarperOne, 2006

Food Films

I had a treatment for a food film in early 2006 called the "Lethal Recipe." A producer and film distributor was interested. They presented the concept to the production company that was, at that time, in production for *Food, Inc*, which meant the fit was not right. Since then, many food films have emerged, and there is now a genre for them, when once it was a rare concept to make an disclosure documentary about the food we eat. Here are a few in a sentence that I've played with in my seminars.

May I Be Frank? If you're *Fed Up* with *Food, Inc* because you get that *Food Matters*, then you're *Hungry for Change*, concerned about the *Future of Food*. You no longer wish to live in a *Fast Food Nation* or *The World According to Monsanto*—seriously, *GMO OMG*—that is full of *Super Size Me* ('s) and has us *Fat, Sick and Nearly Dead*. You know that *King Corn* and *Big Sugar* are *The Human Experiment*, creating *Sweet Misery* and threatening our survival. Confused whether you need to choose *Forks Over Knives*? Go *Simply Raw* and get *Vegucated* without a huge *Food Fight*. If you want to know the *Truth About Food*, then simply *Return to Food*.

WEBSITES

This is a tough one, as there are countless awesome sites, but here are a few you'll love.

www.youngandraw.com: great recipes for raw food enthusiasts and people wanting to do cleanses
www.runningwithnature.com: Mariel Hemingway and Bobby Williams's site
www.mindbodygreen.com: great aggregate site for health-oriented articles
www.laptoplunches.com: over 365 recipe ideas for healthy lunches
www.biodynamics.com: the future of feeding the world and preserving the earth
www.permacultureprinciples.com: brilliant practical ideas on how to feed the world sustainably
www.oprah.com/app/super-soul-sunday: I love the interviews Oprah does in this series of soulicious wisdom
www.TED.com: for a range of inspiring talks on any subject you can think of
www.tut.com/account/register: for the best words of inspiration from the universe

PEOPLE

There are hundreds of people who've inspired me over the years, and influenced, taught, and delighted me on my journey—way too many to mention, but here are the first who come to mind. Vandana Shiva is a quantum physicist and activist for food security and food justice. She is one of the most intelligent, clear, and inspiring voices in the world on how we need to return to food.

Michael Pollen, whose book *In Defence of Food* had my biggest supporters worried my book was already published. His writing is well researched and super sensible.

Mariel Hemingway and Bobby Williams: I'm like their Benjamin Button love child dwarfed by their presence, but I love their company and how they really live and love life.

Stephanie Alexander and Alice Waters, who've done so much for getting kids into the garden, the kitchen and returning to eating real food.

Kris Carr of *Crazy Sexy* fame, who does things with such joy you gotta love her.

Socially Yours

www.instagram.com/sherrystrong1
Twitter: www.twitter.com/sherrystrong
Facebook: www.facebook.com/returntofood
Website: www.returntofood.com
Return to Food Academy: free webinar at www.returntofood.tv

AUTHOR BIOGRAPHY

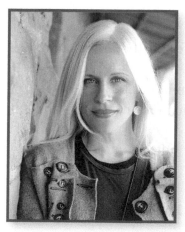

Sherry Strong is a food philosopher, chef and nutritionist. She was the Curator & Co-Founder of the World Wellness Project, Victorian Chair of Nutrition Australia, Melbourne President of Slow Food, a TEDxTokyo 2009 speaker and on the faculty of the Institute of Holistic Nutrition in Vancouver.

Once twice her present size, Sherry dropped 8 dress sizes by hopping off the diet treadmill and taking a holistic, philosophical, loving approach to developing a healthy relationship with food and her body. Her food and nutrition expertise has seen her share these philosophies around the world. Due to demand, she's created the Return to Food Academy, where she teaches people, holistic culinary skills; how to speak professionally on and off camera; and how to create a thriving holistic business as 'Return to Food' coaches, leaders and entrepreneurs.

Sherry lives on Bowen Island on Canada's west coast where she runs retreats, with upcoming holistic adventures for Return to Food Academy graduates in France, India, Australia, Italy and the UK.

- Access to digital bonuses worth over $197.
- Sherry's two (75+ minutes) digital DVDs- The Seven Recipes for Life and The Seven Smoothies for Life, filmed in Australia.
- Calming meditation video filmed at Contemplation Point on Bowen Island.
- Access to five exclusive videos of Conversations with Masters, which features leaders and experts who have inspired Sherry.
- A video and PDF on how to pack a holistic travel kitchen in your suitcase and the Return to Food Eating Out Guide.

The Return to Food Online Program and The Return to Food Academy:

If the material in this book speaks to you in a way in which you would like to learn more or even create an income helping people through a "Return to Food", read on…

Sherry offers an 8 week program based on the philosophies in her book, while also going deeper into the concepts and materials she shares with her clients through lifestyle makeovers worth thousands of dollars. The online program is the prerequisite program for The Return to Food Academy where you can learn to become a Return to Food coach, advocate or leader, by building a thriving business as a holistic entrepreneur in the midst of the most delicious food revolution ever.

Check out www.returntofood.com and www.returntofood.tv

If you are interested in developing a career as a Return to Food coach, leader or entrepreneur go to **www.ReturntoFood.com/Academy** for all the information you need.

Praise for the Return to Food Program:

"I'd like to mention that I did a lot of catching up on the program this weekend as I had a lot of time to myself, and I have to say that I have never ever participated in such a complete program with so much valuable information. I'm so glad to be a part of this. It's really amazing."
Caroline Lambert, Holistic Nutritionist

"I'm really enjoying this outstanding program. I'm loving it and learning so much. Thank you!"
Brenda Brooks, Holistic Nutrition Student

"Finding Sherry and the Return to Food program was quite literally an answer to my prayers for both my life and business. It took me on a nourishing journey mentally, spiritually, emotionally and physically and I have walked away with an undeniable calling to be a part of the Return to Food Movement. Return to Food is and will continue to impact people's relationship with themselves, their food and the environment, and I feel eternally blessed to have found it!"
Chanci Dawn, Certified Holistic Weight Loss Coach

"I'm so glad that I met Sherry earlier this year and found Return to Food. Sherry will leave you feeling inspired about your own wellness journey and excited to help others find their path in a non-judgmental and loving way."
Ashley Joyce, Registered Holistic Nutritionist

"Return to Food takes you on a journey of self-discovery and self-love. You will come out of it with so much love for yourself (and) the world around you… People around you will be declaring: "I'll have what she's having!" Return to Food teaches you how to nourish yourself, not just physically but emotionally, spiritually and mentally as well. It teaches you how to find your way to health and there is no need to measure and read and calculate. Just eat, enjoy, feel great and repeat. I haven't felt this good about myself ever."
Gina Sauer, Return to Food Coach & Academy Student

If you want to get on the path to be a published author by Influence Publishing please go to
www.InfluencePublishing.com

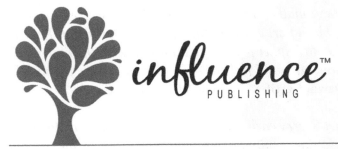

Inspiring books that influence change

More information on our other titles and how to submit your own proposal can be found at
www.InfluencePublishing.com

CPSIA information can be obtained at www.ICGtesting.com
Printed in the USA
LVOW01s1629301014

410929LV00001B/1/P